$22.50

MAR 1 0 1978

Dr. & Mrs. A. Z. Guanzon
1329 ARLINGTON AVENUE
SASKATOON, SASK.
S7H 2Y1

ANAESTHESIA
FOR CARDIAC SURGERY
AND ALLIED PROCEDURES

ANAESTHESIA FOR CARDIAC SURGERY
AND ALLIED PROCEDURES

M. A. BRANTHWAITE
MD MRCP FFARCS

Consultant Physician and Anaesthetist, Brompton Hospital
(National Heart and Chest Hospitals)
Honorary Senior Lecturer, Cardiothoracic Institute, London

with a contribution by
D. J. HATCH FFARCS

Consultant Anaesthetist, Hospital for Sick Children
Great Ormond Street, London

foreword by
M. K. SYKES MA FFARCS

Professor of Clinical Anaesthesia
Royal Postgraduate Medical School, London

BLACKWELL SCIENTIFIC PUBLICATIONS
OXFORD LONDON EDINBURGH MELBOURNE

© 1977 Blackwell Scientific Publications
Osney Mead, Oxford OX2 0EL
8 John Street, London WC1N 2ES
9 Forrest Road, Edinburgh EH1 2QH
P.O. Box 9, North Balwyn, Victoria, Australia

ISBN 0 632 00369 3

First published 1977

British Library Cataloguing in Publication Data

Branthwaite, Margaret Annie
    Anaesthesia for cardiac surgery, and allied procedures
    1. Heart—Surgery   2. Anesthesia
    I. Title
    617'.967'412   RD598

ISBN 0-632-00369-3

Distributed in the U.S.A. by
J. B. Lippincott Company, Philadelphia
and in Canada by
J. B. Lippincott Company of Canada Ltd, Toronto

Set in Monophoto Times

Printed and bound in Great Britain by
Butler & Tanner Ltd, Frome and London

DEDICATED TO D.A.B.

CONTENTS

FOREWORD

The development of closed, and later, open heart surgery has had two major effects on the practice of medicine. In the first place, it has opened up therapeutic possibilities for a number of conditions which were previously considered untreatable. The second, and possibly more important effect, is that it has stimulated a great deal of clinical and experimental research in the fields of physiology, biochemistry, haematology, immunology and bioengineering. Although some of this research has been concerned with problems which are specific to cardiac surgery, much of it has been more fundamental in nature and hence has been of more general application.

Anaesthetists have played a prominent role in these developments, not only in seeking answers to the immediate problems posed by the patient, but also in communicating this new knowledge to their colleagues. The establishment of resuscitation services for the treatment of respiratory and cardiac arrest and the development of respiratory and intensive care units are but two examples of the way in which knowledge gained in the operating theatre has been applied for the benefit of all our patients.

This process is still continuing. For example, recent developments in bedside catheterisation procedures which permit repeated measurements of left atrial pressure have now been widely applied to the treatment of the circulatory disturbances of shock and other conditions encountered in the intensive care unit. It thus becomes apparent that all anaesthetists should have some experience of anaesthesia for cardiac surgery and that those more deeply involved should communicate their knowledge to others.

Dr Branthwaite is the ideal person to carry out this latter task. Trained both as a physician and as an anaesthetist, she has been closely involved with acute cardiological problems and with anaesthesia for cardiac surgery. She has also made notable contributions to research in both of these fields. She has now produced an excellent monograph, critical, concise, well-balanced yet comprehensive and always based on firm physiological foundations. It should be read by all those who are concerned with cardiovascular problems, either in the operating theatre or intensive care unit.

London 1977   M. K. Sykes

PREFACE

Cardiac surgery has advanced rapidly in the last twenty-five years and anaesthetic practice associated with it has changed to a comparable degree. New concepts, new techniques, new drugs and new apparatus introduce improvements or pose new problems and no textbook can be comprehensive or up to date for long. Therefore this text, rather than being aimed specifically at those who specialise in anaesthesia for cardiac surgery, is intended instead for those who are faced with the practical aspects of the subject for the first time and those who wish to amplify their knowledge in preparation for the postgraduate examinations.

The content is didactic rather than discursive and the principles of physiology, pathology and therapeutics which govern anaesthesia for cardiac surgery have been given as much emphasis as the choice of anaesthetic technique. This approach is based on the belief that a clear understanding of the problems presented by an individual patient is of greater importance than the detail of the technique selected. The methods recommended reflect current practice at the Brompton Hospital but alternatives are discussed where necessary. A selection of further reading is given at the end of each chapter, references being grouped under subject headings so that the interested reader can explore a particular topic in depth rather than refer to individual points identified within the text.

The author is greatly indebted to many colleagues at the Brompton Hospital who read and commented on parts of the manuscript, particularly Dr M. J. H. Scallan who read the entire text and made a number of helpful suggestions.

Dr D. J. Hatch of the Hospital for Sick Children, Great Ormond Street, contributed the chapter on anaesthesia for cardiac surgery in the first year of life and Dr R. D. Bradley of St Thomas' Hospital supplied a number of the illustrations and kindly commented on the early chapters.

Finally, I am particularly grateful to Professor M. K. Sykes who not only read and commented constructively on the entire text but also contributed a generous foreword. It is a great pleasure to acknowledge the help of so many friends and colleagues.

London 1977   M. A. Branthwaite

CHAPTER 1

APPLIED PHYSIOLOGY OF THE HEART AND CIRCULATION

Intrinsic regulatory mechanisms
Heterometric response
Homeometric regulation
Extrinsic regulatory mechanisms
Implications of impaired cardiac function

Abnormalities of intrinsic mechanisms
Heterometric response
Homeometric response
External regulatory mechanisms in heart failure
Integrated circulation
Circulation in heart failure

The normal heart is regulated by a number of mechanisms which combine to allow considerable variation in performance. It is customary to classify these mechanisms as 'intrinsic' or 'extrinsic', the intrinsic group being fundamental properties of cardiac muscle, while the extrinsic factors are the effects of neurological and hormonal stimuli.

INTRINSIC REGULATORY MECHANISMS

Heterometric response

The most important of the intrinsic properties is the heterometric response or Frank-Starling mechanism. The Frank-Starling 'law' states that 'up to a point, cardiac output rises as ventricular filling is increased', but this is no more than an application of the more fundamental statement that the force of contraction is proportional to the initial fibre length (which for the ventricle, is end-diastolic fibre length).

At first sight, the terms of this relationship bear little relevance to clinical practice, largely because neither can be measured easily. In spite of this difficulty, manipulation of the heterometric response forms the basis for management of many types of circulatory failure, and therefore it is necessary to digress to explore how this important relationship is evaluated in clinical terms.

Although the force of myocardial contraction cannot be measured easily, the work of the heart is readily appreciated, each ventricle generating both flow and pressure within the corresponding vascular bed. For clinical purposes, it is convenient to discuss cardiac performance in terms of either stroke

1

work or stroke volume. Stroke volume is the simplest variable to consider, but stroke work is sometimes a more meaningful concept particularly in heart failure. Stroke work is expressed mathematically as the product of stroke volume times the pressure gradient through which that volume of blood has been moved, i.e. for the left ventricle, stroke work equals:

stroke volume × (mean arterial − ventricular end-diastolic pressure).

In the same way that stroke volume or stroke work is often used in the clinical context instead of force of contraction, terms of more immediate practical significance are selected in preference to 'initial fibre length'. It is entirely reasonable to assume that the initial (end-diastolic) length of ventricular fibres bears a direct relationship to ventricular end-diastolic volume, but this too is a variable which is difficult to determine. It is much easier to measure intravascular pressure, but the assumption that changes in end-diastolic *pressure* always reflect comparable changes in ventricular end-diastolic *volume* is questionable. Although ventricular end-diastolic pressure and volume may be linearly related over a wide range in the normal heart, a fibrous, overstretched ventricle is relatively non-compliant. Quite small increments of volume (and hence in end-diastolic fibre length) cause relatively large changes in ventricular end-diastolic pressure. In these circumstances end-diastolic pressure is a poor reflection of ventricular filling. An additional problem is introduced if mean atrial pressure is monitored instead of ventricular end-diastolic pressure. There is close correlation between these two variables in the normal heart but there may be a considerable discrepancy between them in the presence of chronic cardiac disease. There may also be a considerable discrepancy between the two atrial pressures (p. 5), and relating changes in *left* ventricular performance to mean *right* atrial (central venous) pressure ignore this distinction. It is apparent from this analysis that the clinically useful description of the heterometric response in terms of stroke work or volume related to central venous pressure is derived from the fundamental property by a number of assumptions which are invalid in some circumstances (Table 1.1).

Table 1.1   Derivation of the relationship between stroke volume and central venous pressure through a chain of assumptions from the fundamental property.

Force of contraction	Initial fibre length
Stroke work	Ventricular end-diastolic volume
Stroke volume	Ventricular end-diastolic pressure
	Mean atrial pressure
	Central venous pressure

Homeometric regulation

There are two other intrinsic regulatory properties in addition to the heterometric (Frank-Starling) mechanism.

If the normal heart is exposed to an abrupt increase in peripheral resistance, the stroke volume falls for a few beats but then returns to its previous value without any change in end-diastolic fibre length, and without the operation of any reflex neurological or hormonally mediated compensatory mechanism. In other words, the myocardium has adjusted to generate a greater work load (more pressure) without invoking either the Frank-Starling mechanism or any external regulatory influence. This intrinsic property is known as the Anrep effect.

A similar adjustment, known as the Bowditch effect, permits the heart to beat at a greater rate without reduction in stroke volume, again without encroaching on either the heterometric response or any external mechanism.

EXTRINSIC REGULATORY MECHANISMS

In the intact circulation, the myocardium is influenced by the autonomic nervous system and by the action of circulating hormones, in particular adrenaline and noradrenaline. Stimulation of the sympathetic system augments the force of contraction (inotropic effect) and increases the heart rate (chronotropic action). These are both beta-one sympathomimetic effects and endogenous sympathetic stimulation leads to a simultaneous increase in both rate and force of contraction; some separation of the chronotropic and inotropic properties can be achieved pharmacologically by selective beta-adrenergic agonists or blocking agents.

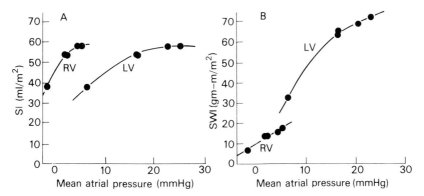

Figure 1.1 Ventricular function curves for the two sides of the heart. The relationship between (a) stroke index (SI) or (b) stroke work index (SWI) and mean atrial pressure (MAP) in a patient aged 20 suffering from acute glomerulonephritis. Pressure measurements were referred to zero at the sternal angle. RV = right ventricle; LV = left ventricle. Reproduced from Bradley *et al.*, 1971, by permission of the Editor, *Cardiovascular Research*.

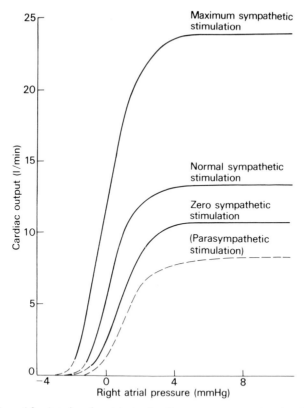

Figure 1.2 A series of ventricular function curves representing the effects of autonomic stimulation on the heart. From Guyton *et al.*, 1973, reproduced by permission
of W. B. Saunders Co.

Stimulation of the parasympathetic system results in bradycardia. There
is also a slight negative inotropic effect, i.e. the force of contraction is depressed
by vagal stimulation, but this is usually of trivial importance. In a healthy
subject at rest, the myocardium is influenced predominantly by the parasympathetic system, but sympathomimetic activity assumes greater importance
when an increase in output is required, e.g. during exercise.

There is always considerable interplay between the intrinsic and extrinsic
regulatory mechanisms, exemplified by considering the effects of sympathomimetic agents on the heterometric response. Within the limitations discussed already, the heterometric response can be described in terms of the
relationship between either stroke work or stroke volume and mean atrial
pressure. The line relating these two variables is called a ventricular function
curve (Fig. 1.1), and a whole series of curves can be constructed which
represent the performance of the heart under varying degrees of autonomic
nervous activity. Thus sympathomimetic stimulation, which augments con-

tractility, moves the function curve upwards and to the left, whereas negative inotropic agents depress and flatten the curve (Fig. 1.2).

IMPLICATIONS OF IMPAIRED CARDIAC FUNCTION

The term cardiac failure can be defined in a number of ways: clinically, by the association of a group of characteristic symptoms and signs, or physiologically, in terms of some measurable abnormality. Although the latter approach is more logical, it is impossible to define 'contractility' in terms of a single, easily measured response, and a number of methods have been devised, each evaluating a different aspect of cardiac function.
They include:

1   The timing of events during the cardiac cycle.
2   The haemodynamic response to stress (exercise, pacing, or induced changes in blood pressure).
3   The ability of the ventricle to empty during systole.
4   The velocity of muscle fibre shortening.
5   The rate of rise of ventricular pressure.
6   The response of the myocardium to changes in fibre length.

Unfortunately, there are both theoretical and practical disadvantages to several of these techniques and the demonstration of an abnormal response is sometimes of limited clinical significance. In practice, it is often more convenient to consider how impairment of cardiac function interferes with the normal regulatory mechanisms described in the preceding section.

ABNORMALITIES OF INTRINSIC MECHANISMS

Heterometric response

It has been shown that the performance of the normal heart can be described by a family of ventricular function curves relating either stroke work or stroke volume to mean atrial pressure. Increased contractility moves the curve upwards and to the left, whereas depression of function, by drugs or disease, lowers and flattens the curve. When heart failure is very severe, there is a fixed low output which is independent of changes in filling pressure (Fig. 1.3).

In some circumstances, the function of one side of the heart is impaired to a greater degree than the other; a good example is acute myocardial infarction which often involves only the left ventricle. This situation is illustrated in Fig. 1.4 in which it is apparent that the left ventricular function curve is depressed and flattened to a greater degree than that for the right. The same stroke volume is ejected from the two sides of the heart, but the filling pressure on the left greatly exceeds that on the right. Pulmonary oedema occurs when the rate at which fluid leaves the pulmonary capillaries exceeds the capacity for fluid removal of the pulmonary lymphatics; this usually occurs when the mean hydrostatic pressure in the pulmonary capillaries

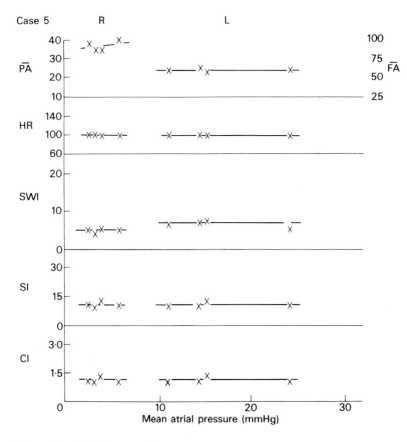

Figure 1.3 The influence of changes in atrial pressure on a number of haemodynamic variables in a man of 56 suffering from myocardial infarction complicated by pulmonary embolism. All pressure measurements were referred to zero at the sternal angle. R = right heart; L = left heart; $\overline{PA}$ and $\overline{FA}$ = mean pulmonary and femoral arterial pressures; HR = heart rate; SWI = stroke work index; SI = stroke index; CI = cardiac index. Reproduced from Bradley *et al.*, 1970, by permission of The American Heart Association, Inc.

exceeds approximately 28 mm Hg (3·7 kPa). It is apparent from Fig. 1.4 that pulmonary oedema will be generated in this patient at right atrial pressures above 4 mm Hg (0·5 kPa) when the corresponding left atrial (and hence pul-

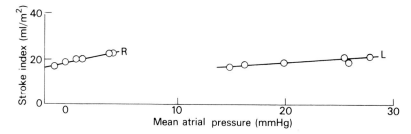

Figure 1.4 Ventricular function curves recorded from a patient aged 56 years suffering from myocardial infarction. The symbols, source and acknowledgements are as in Fig. 1.3.

monary capillary) pressure will exceed 25 mm Hg (3·3 kPa); in addition, relatively minor alterations in right atrial pressure will be associated with considerable alterations in left atrial pressure.

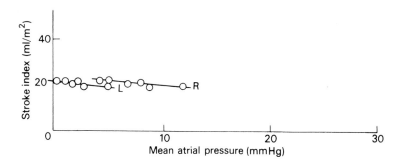

Figure 1.5 Ventricular function curves recorded from a patient aged 49 years suffering from acute, massive pulmonary embolism. The symbols are as in Fig. 1.3.

A different situation exists when right ventricular function is impaired to a greater degree than the left. In the case illustrated in Fig. 1.5, the right atrial pressure exceeds that on the left throughout the range studied; filling of the left ventricle, reflected by the left atrial pressure, will be inadequate unless the right atrial pressure is well above the normal range.

As a general rule, the higher of the two atrial pressures relates to the ventricle which is under greatest stress; management during cardiac surgery therefore requires that both atrial pressures be monitored, particularly when there is likely to be a discrepancy between the performance of the two sides of the heart.

Homeometric response

The failing heart is unable to compensate for either an increase in the resistance against which it ejects (increased after-load), or for an increase in heart
rate, and the stroke volume falls in both cases. When the after-load increases,
a smaller stroke volume is ejected against a greater resistance and the stroke
work may be unchanged. However, the genesis of pressure is often of less
value physiologically than the maintenance of flow, and therefore it is important to protect the failing ventricle from extreme elevation of the corresponding arterial pressure.

EXTERNAL REGULATORY MECHANISMS IN HEART FAILURE

Stimulation of the sympathetic system and catecholamine secretion from the
adrenal medulla augment the performance of the normal heart and are involved in the myocardial response to increased demand, e.g. on exercise.
When ventricular function is impaired, the efficacy of the intrinsic properties
of the heart is gradually eroded; any improvement in cardiac performance
is increasingly dependent on sympathomimetic stimulation until ultimately,
cardiac output at rest is maintained by sympathetic drive. When this situation
exists, the cardiac output is low, it cannot increase in response to exercise
or stress, and it will fall even further, perhaps disastrously, if beta-adrenergic
blocking agents are used. With this degree of heart failure, there are no
reserves of cardiac function and relatively slight myocardial depression
caused by hypoxia, hypercarbia or anaesthetic drugs can lead to circulatory
failure.

THE INTEGRATED CIRCULATION

The foregoing discussion has concentrated on the performance of the heart
and how this is regulated in health and disease. Myocardial contractility
is, however, only one variable in a complex interplay of control mechanisms which determine the function of the circulation as a whole; other
factors of importance are peripheral vascular (arteriolar) resistance, venous
tone, blood volume and its composition, and the state of the pulmonary vasculature. When the heart is failing, these other variables must be
adjusted to minimise, as far as possible, deleterious effects on circulatory
function.

CIRCULATION IN HEART FAILURE

The importance of sympathetic stimulation as a means of supporting the failing myocardium has been described already but sympathetic activity also influences peripheral vascular resistance and venous tone. If the cardiac output falls abruptly, baroceptor stimulation provokes a reflex increase in sympathetic activity which improves myocardial performance, increases venous tone and causes peripheral arteriolar constriction. The increase in venous tone results in a transfer of blood from the peripheral capacitance vessels into the central circulation (great veins, heart and lungs), and ventricular filling pressure rises as a result. Until myocardial failure is extreme or unless the ventricle is already overfilled, an increase in filling pressure will augment the force of contraction by operation of the heterometric response, so tending to restore the cardiac output to normal. If the output remains low in spite of venoconstriction, peripheral arteriolar constriction occurs as well, so restricting blood flow to non-essential tissues and maintaining the arterial blood pressure even though the cardiac output is reduced. Tissue oxygen uptake continues unaltered, but mixed venous blood is abnormally desaturated because overall blood flow is diminished.

If the output falls more gradually, changes in vascular tone are less prominent and ventricular filling is augmented by an increase in blood volume which is brought about by the renal retention of salt and water. The stimuli which initiate fluid retention are incompletely understood but include baroceptor impulses from the great veins, pulmonary circulation and the arterial system, changes in renal blood flow and haemodynamics, and an increased secretion of aldosterone. The distribution of the increased blood volume between the pulmonary and peripheral vessels depends on the relative performance of the two sides of the heart and this, in turn, is responsible for the symptoms and signs which result.

The combination of pulmonary or systemic venous engorgement and a reduced cardiac output results in a number of sequelae affecting other tissues and organs which are described in Chapter 2.

REFERENCES

PHYSIOLOGY

BRADLEY R. D., JENKINS, B. S. & BRANTHWAITE, M. A. (1970) The influence of atrial pressure on cardiac performance following myocardial infarction complicated by shock. *Circulation* **42**, 827.

BRADLEY R. D., JENKINS B. S. & BRANTHWAITE M. A. (1971) Myocardial function in acute glomerulonephritis. *Cardiovascular Research* **5**, 223.

BRAUNWALD E. (1965) The control of ventricular function in man. *British Heart Journal* **27**, 1.

BRAUNWALD E. (1971) Editorial 'On the difference between the heart's output and its contractile state'. *Circulation* **43**, 171.

Ciba Symposium 24 (new series) (1974) *The Physiological Basis of Starling's Law of the Heart.* American Elsevier Publishing, New York.

GUYTON A. C., JONES C. E. & COLEMAN T. G. (1973) *Circulatory Physiology: Cardiac Output and its Regulation.* W. B. Saunders, Philadelphia.

HARRISON A. H. (1975) Contractile basis of heart failure. In *Modern Trends in Cardiology 3*, Ed. M. F. Oliver, p. 182. Butterworth, London.

KELMAN G. R. (1971). *Applied Cardiovascular Physiology.* Butterworth, London.

NAYLER W. G. (1975) The ionic basis of contractility, relaxation, and cardiac failure. In *Modern Trends in Cardiology 3*, Ed. M. F. Oliver, p. 154. Butterworth, London.

OLSON C. B. & WAUD D. R. (1970) On looking at electrical activity of heart muscle. *Anesthesiology* **33**, 520.

RUSSELL W. J. (1974) Central venous pressure in cardiovascular dynamics. Part I of *Central Venous Pressure: its clinical use and role in cardiovascular dynamics.* Butterworth, London.

SIEGEL J. H. (1969) The myocardial contractile state and its role in the response to anaesthesia and surgery. *Anesthesiology* **30**, 519.

TY SMITH N. & HOFFMAN J. I. E. (1969) Evaluation of the circulation—pulmonary and otherwise—in man. *Anesthesiology* **30**, 589.

ASSESSMENT OF MYOCARDIAL FUNCTION

KREULEN T. H., BOVE A. A., MCDONOUGH M. T., SANDS M. J. & SPANN J. F. (1975) The evaluation of left ventricular function in man: a comparison of methods. *Circulation* **51**, 677.

MITCHELL J. H., WILDENTHAL K., VAN DEN BOS G. C., LINDEN R. J., SNOW H. M. & TAYLOR S. H. (1972) Symposium on 'Problems in measurement of myocardial contractility'. *Proceedings of the Royal Society of Medicine* **65**, 542.

REITAN J. A., TY SMITH N., BORISON V. S. & KADIS L. B. (1972) The cardiac pre-ejection period: a correlate of peak ascending aortic blood flow acceleration. *Anesthesiology* **36**, 76.

ROSS J. Jr & PETERSON K. L. (1973) On the assessment of cardiac inotropic state. *Circulation* **47**, 435.

TOMLIN P. J., DUCK F., MCNULTY M. & GREEN C. D. (1975) A comparison of methods of evaluating myocardial contractility. *Canadian Anaesthetists' Society Journal* **22**, 436.

CHAPTER 2

SEQUELAE OF CARDIAC DISEASE

Pulmonary venous congestion
Abnormalities of pulmonary function
Pulmonary vascular disease
Systemic venous congestion
Other manifestations of cardiac disease
Dysrhythmias
Embolism
Bacterial endocarditis and rheumatic carditis
Circulatory failure and cardiac arrest

Specific features of congenital heart disease
Effects of drug therapy
Digitalis
Diuretics
Anticoagulants
β-adrenergic blocking agents
Hypotensive drugs
Sedatives

PULMONARY VENOUS CONGESTION

Pulmonary venous congestion is a sequel to disorders of the left side of the heart, including mitral and aortic valve disease as well as defects of left ventricular muscle. The cardinal symptom is dyspnoea, initially only on exertion, but eventually occurring at rest. Exertional dyspnoea is customarily classified into four categories:

Grade I   Dyspnoea on more than average activity, e.g. running, or walking up hills.
Grade II   Dyspnoea on ordinary activity, e.g. climbing two flights of stairs.
Grade III Dyspnoea on less than ordinary activity, e.g. walking slowly on the level.
Grade IV   Total incapacity.

Dyspnoea caused by pulmonary venous congestion is exacerbated when the intrathoracic blood volume is increased by recumbency (orthopnoea), and attacks of paroxysmal nocturnal dyspnoea are common for the same reason. Distension of bronchopulmonary anastomoses leads to congestion of bronchial vessels which in turn causes bronchial mucosal swelling, and hence peripheral airways obstruction—'cardiac asthma'. Bronchial mucus is secreted in excess but tends to be thick and sticky unlike the thin frothy sputum of pulmonary oedema. Unless the pulmonary vasculature is abnormal, oedema develops when the hydrostatic pressure in the pulmonary capillaries exceeds approximately 28 m Hg (3·7 kPa). It is characterised by the expectoration of pink, frothy sputum although sputum production may be minimal in the early stages when a dry cough is a prominent feature.

11

Abnormalities of pulmonary function

Conventional tests of lung function reveal a decrease in both the vital capacity and total lung capacity, and the ratio of forced expiratory volume in one second to forced vital capacity is reduced if bronchial narrowing is present. Pulmonary compliance is diminished and airway resistance high, so that the work required to move a given volume of air is greatly increased. Measurements of the transfer factor can be misleading because the ability to transfer oxygen or carbon monoxide across the pulmonary alveolar–capillary membrane depends on both the pulmonary capillary volume (V_c) and the 'membrane component' (D_m). In the early stages of pulmonary venous congestion (e.g. early mitral stenosis), the increase in pulmonary capillary blood volume may more than offset any interference with gas transfer caused by maldistribution or true abnormalities of diffusion, and the measured value for the transfer factor is then supranormal at rest. However, it fails to increase normally on exercise and is decreased even at rest when pulmonary venous congestion is severe, or if pulmonary vascular disease develops (p. 13).

The distribution of blood flow within the lungs is also abnormal. In a healthy upright subject, pulmonary blood flow is distributed preferentially to the bases of the lungs but this preferential basal perfusion is lost when pulmonary venous congestion occurs. Diversion of blood to the upper lobes results and is apparent radiologically as an increase in the diameter of the upper lobe veins. This appearance precedes the development of pulmonary oedema. Kerley B lines may also be seen relatively early. They represent distended pulmonary lymphatics and septal oedema, and are best seen in the lower zones at the periphery of the lung fields.

Bronchial narrowing distorts the distribution of alveolar ventilation, and the combination of disturbances in both perfusion and ventilation results in a considerable increase in physiological dead space and in the shunt effect. It might be anticipated that this inefficiency of gas exchange would lead to hypoxia and hypercarbia, but in the majority of patients the minute volume is increased to such an extent that the arterial carbon dioxide tension is low. Hypoxia cannot be corrected without augmenting the inspired oxygen concentration, and low arterial oxygen and carbon dioxide tensions are therefore the characteristic findings in air-breathing patients suffering from pulmonary venous congestion or pulmonary oedema.

There are probably several stimuli contributing to the increase in minute volume: arterial hypoxaemia, stretch receptors in the walls of the great vessels, atria and in the lungs, and possibly relative ischaemia of the respiratory centre. Tachypnoea is obvious, and the tidal volume is generally increased too although this is usually less noticeable. The respiratory workload is particularly great because of the need to sustain a high minute volume when pulmonary compliance is low and airway resistance is high; ultimately, the increased oxygen demand caused by the effort of hyperventilation is greater than the oxygen uptake which results from it.

When pulmonary oedema is severe, and particularly if the cardiac output is low as well, the arterial carbon dioxide tension rises. This is relatively uncommon and does not have the same significance as hypercapnia in patients suffering from chronic pulmonary disease. The administration of oxygen in high concentrations does not lead to carbon dioxide narcosis when hypercapnia accompanies pulmonary oedema, and respiratory depressant drugs are not contraindicated.

Cheyne-Stokes respiration is sometimes a feature of left ventricular failure. This cyclic variation in tidal volume occurs when there is a prolonged lung to brain circulation time and therefore a lag between changes in alveolar ventilation and the consequent alteration of carbon dioxide tension in blood reaching the respiratory centre (Fig. 2.1). The cycle length is equal to approximately twice the lung to brain circulation time and may be 90 seconds or more in severe left ventricular failure. Cheyne-Stokes respiration occurs more readily if the respiratory centre is relatively unresponsive to carbon dioxide, for example because of cerebrovascular disease or if opiates have been given. The arterial carbon dioxide tension is always low when Cheyne-Stokes respiration occurs as a result of left ventricular failure.

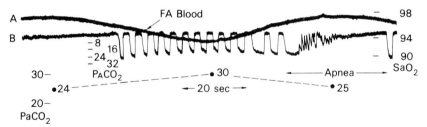

Figure 2.1 Changes in the saturation of femoral arterial blood (A), the expired carbon dioxide tension (B), and the arterial carbon dioxide tension during Cheyne-Stokes respiration. From Lange & Hecht, 1962, by permission of the Editor, Journal of Clinical Investigation.

Pulmonary vascular disease

The pulmonary arterial pressure is slightly elevated in the early stages of pulmonary venous congestion, reflecting nothing more than the abnormally high pressures in the left heart and pulmonary veins. The pulmonary vascular resistance

$$\frac{\text{mean pulmonary arterial} - \text{mean left atrial pressure}}{\text{pulmonary blood flow (i.e. cardiac output)}}$$

is normal. The pulmonary vasculature is relatively normal in histological appearance and oedema fluid can pass readily through the thin walls of the pulmonary capillaries. Frank extravasation of blood may occur and result in haemoptysis, although blood in the sputum can also originate from the congested bronchial mucosa, especially during attacks of bronchitis which are common when the lungs and bronchi are engorged. If the condition remains unrelieved, irreversible anatomical changes develop within the lungs. There is haemosiderosis, fibrosis and thickening of the alveolar walls, the pulmonary venules and small pulmonary veins show intimal fibrosis and medial thickening, there is medial thickening and intimal proliferation in the pulmonary arterioles and small muscular arteries, and the larger subdivisions of the pulmonary artery are dilated and atheromatous. The pulmonary vascular resistance is increased and the pulmonary arterial pressure markedly elevated; this leads to right ventricular hypertrophy, and ultimately to right heart failure.

Table 2.1 Pulmonary function in a patient with long-standing mitral valve disease. Pulmonary hypertension had been documented 14 years before these results were obtained.

	Predicted	*Result*
Forced expiratory volume in 1 second (ml)	2600	675
Forced vital capacity (ml)	3740	2000
Total lung capacity (ml)	5910	6130
Transfer factor for carbon monoxide (mmol $min^{-1} kPa^{-1}$)	8·67	5·93

Pulmonary function deteriorates at the same time. There is often a long history of recurrent attacks of wheezy bronchitis, and lung function tests reveal severe airways obstruction which may be largely irreversible (Table 2.1). The total lung capacity and functional residual capacity are variable, depending upon the relative importance of airways obstruction, pulmonary fibrosis, venous engorgement and vascular obliteration. Deranged pulmonary function may be more important than pulmonary venous congestion as a cause of dyspnoea, and both cardiac catheterisation and detailed testing of lung function may be required to assess the relative importance of cardiac and pulmonary disease. These patients are very likely to develop respiratory insufficiency after operation, and unlike those with early pulmonary venous congestion, hypercapnia occurs easily so that unrestricted oxygen therapy and respiratory depressant drugs can both be dangerous.

These changes take time to develop and are the classical features of long-standing mitral stenosis. Other cardiac disorders can give rise to similar pulmonary pathology, but the natural history of the primary disease is often shorter and the pulmonary and pulmonary vascular changes are therefore less apparent.

SYSTEMIC VENOUS CONGESTION

Unlike pulmonary venous congestion which causes severe functional derangements which are of considerable importance during and after anaesthesia, systemic venous congestion is symptomatic of the severity of the disease but has much less specific anaesthetic significance. The presence of the classical signs of right ventricular failure implies that there are no reserves of cardiac function; the cardiac output is low although generally adequate for the resting patient. Abnormalities of renal function are common and the blood urea is often elevated. The liver is enlarged and jaundice and abnormal liver function tests may be detected, e.g. a prolonged prothrombin time in the absence of anticoagulant therapy. Abnormalities of hepatic function are particularly likely to occur when the venous distension is pulsatile as in tricuspid incompetence. Many patients in heart failure are anorexic, and some develop abdominal pain and nausea which may be caused by hepatic engorgement, congestion of the gastric mucosa, or the effects of drugs. Cachexia is a late feature, seen most frequently in patients with long-standing valvular disease, especially those with pulmonary hypertension. These patients are underweight, malnourished and have evidence of parenchymal disease of both the liver and kidneys. The significance of this lies in the sensivity which they show to anaesthetic agents; drug absorption, transport and excretion may all be abnormal and these points should be borne in mind, especially when premedication is being prescribed.

OTHER MANIFESTATIONS OF CARDIAC DISEASE

Dysrhythmias

Rhythm disorders are an integral part of heart disease and often complicate cardiac surgery. They may be present preoperatively and some are particularly associated with specific conditions, e.g. atrial fibrillation with mitral stenosis. During and after surgery, mechanical, biochemical and pharmacological stimuli can all precipitate rhythm changes and some hearts are more 'irritable' than others, irrespective of the underlying pathology. Rhythm changes are important because they often cause an abrupt deterioration in circulatory function which, if unchecked, will aggravate myocardial failure and may herald the onset of even more serious dysrhythmias. Sometimes, however, the rhythm change is self-limiting.

Embolism

Systemic embolism is the other major hazard of rhythm changes and is particularly likely to occur in patients experiencing paroxysmal attacks of atrial fibrillation. Clot forms in the dilated atria during episodes of fibrillation and is discharged into the circulation when coordinated atrial contraction returns. Clot can also form within the heart on damaged or non-epithelialised surfaces, for example after myocardial infarction or on prosthetic valves and patches; systemic embolism can then occur without any change of rhythm. Sometimes a single large clot is thrown off, but commonly there are showers of small emboli which affect several organs simultaneously. A rare cause of systemic embolism is left atrial myxoma. This tumour is generally benign and often pedunculated. Signs of variable mitral valve disease are associated with fever, anaemia and a raised ESR; complete recovery usually follows removal of the tumour.

Pulmonary emboli are likely to arise from blood clot in the vessels of the legs and pelvis in patients who are immobile and bed-ridden; subsequent infarction is particularly likely to occur in those with pulmonary venous congestion. Pulmonary infarction also follows thrombosis within the pulmonary circulation which may occur when the vessels are dilated and atheromatous.

Bacterial endocarditis and rheumatic carditis

Infection is liable to develop within the heart wherever there is an abnormal valve or surface although it is rarely associated with some common lesions, e.g. atrial septal defect. The infection is generally subacute and presents insidiously with malaise, low-grade fever and anaemia. Systemic embolism can occur if the vegetations fragment but much of the organ pathology such as microscopic haematuria and impaired renal function is caused by the deposition of immune complexes. There may be abrupt haemodynamic deterioration, for example if infection causes perforation of a valve cusp, and emergency valve replacement may be necessary before a full course of chemotherapy has been completed. Surgery may also be required in the presence of sepsis if a prosthetic valve is infected; these can rarely be sterilised with systemic antibiotics. Such patients present particular problems during anaesthesia: not only are they anaemic, febrile and in cardiac or even circulatory failure, but surgery is hazardous because the tissues are friable and do not hold sutures well.

Similar problems attend operation in the presence of active rheumatic carditis. It is occasionally necessary to repair or replace a severely damaged valve before the disease is quiescent although this is avoided whenever possible. The tissues are friable, conduction defects are common, and pericarditis is an almost inevitable accompaniment. This causes numerous vascular adhesions which are often the source of troublesome haemorrhage. Corticosteroid supplements may be required during anaesthesia because these drugs are often used to treat active rheumatic carditis.

Circulatory failure and cardiac arrest

Circulatory failure is the obvious end point of cardiac disease. It can occur suddenly following myocardial infarction, pulmonary embolism or the onset of a dysrhythmia, or may develop gradually over days or months. It is difficult to provide a precise definition, but the term implies that the condition is deteriorating rather than stable, that the vital organs are inadequately perfused, even when the patient is at rest, and ultimately, that there is systemic hypotension and peripheral vasoconstriction. Death is inevitable unless it is possible to bring about a major improvement in some aspect of cardiac function. This may entail emergency surgery in an unprepared patient and whatever the nature of the operation, the risks associated with anaesthesia, the procedure itself, and the postoperative period are all very high. Points of particular importance are dealt with in subsequent chapters where specific conditions are discussed.

Cardiac arrest can occur as a terminal event after a prolonged period of circulatory failure or may happen suddenly in a patient who was previously well. Some conditions such as severe aortic stenosis and acute myocardial ischaemia are associated with a particularly high incidence of unexpected cardiac arrest. Management depends to some extent upon the circumstances of the arrest but the principles are always the same: adequate support of the circulation, efficient ventilation, correction of biochemical abnormalities, and specific measures to restore an effective heart beat. Special features of the practical management of cardiac arrest during cardiac surgery are discussed on pp. 90 and 103.

SPECIFIC FEATURES OF CONGENITAL HEART DISEASE

The preceding sections have dealt largely with the sequelae of acquired cardiac disease. Many of the points discussed apply equally well to patients suffering from congenital heart disease, but there are some congenital lesions which warrant separate consideration, in particular, those in which there is an abnormal communication between the pulmonary and systemic circulations. Such a communication permits blood to flow from right to left or vice versa, the direction of flow depending on the relative resistance of the outflow tract and vascular bed on the two sides of the circulation. Arterialised blood reaches the right heart or pulmonary artery (left to right shunt) when there is an uncomplicated patent ductus arteriosus, atrial or ventricular septal defect. The pulmonary blood flow is increased and is commonly between two and three times that in the systemic circulation. When the left to right communication is at atrial level, the shunt is between two relatively low pressure chambers. The pressure in the pulmonary circulation is increased only slightly in spite of the considerable increase in blood flow through it. In ventricular septal defect and patent ductus arteriosus, the shunt flow is derived from a high pressure source (left ventricle or aorta), and the pulmonary arterial pressure is therefore elevated considerably. Sometimes the shunt is of such magnitude that pulmonary oedema occurs in infancy and corrective or pallia- tive surgery is required if the child is to survive (pp. 164 and 173), but many patients with these lesions reach adult life and may be symptom-free for a number of years.

Chronic exposure of the pulmonary circulation to a high flow, particularly at a high pressure, elicits secondary changes within the pulmonary vascu- lature which consist of arterial wall hypertrophy and an increase in pul- monary vascular resistance. This eventually limits the flow through the shunt and may even reverse the direction so that blood flows from right to left and the patient develops central cyanosis (Eisenmenger syndrome). Initially, the increase in pulmonary vascular resistance is reversible, the pulmonary arterial pressure falling if high concentrations of oxygen are given. Closure of the shunt at this stage prevents the development of irreversible pulmonary vascu- lar changes. Ultimately, the pulmonary vascular resistance is so high that the shunt flow is predominantly from right to left, even at rest, and the pul- monary arterial pressure remains elevated when oxygen is given. The condi- tion is then inoperable and closure of the shunt will cause right ventricular failure which proves rapidly fatal.

Changes within the pulmonary circulation occur more slowly if the shunt is at atrial level and the pulmonary arterial pressure is elevated initially to a lesser degree. These patients may remain symptom-free until late middle- age although pulmonary plethora predisposes them to recurrent attacks of bronchitis. Ultimately they present either with dyspnoea or with right heart failure, often precipitated by the onset of atrial fibrillation. Pulmonary func- tion is generally abnormal by then, most patients showing features of chronic obstructive airways disease; respiratory difficulties are common postopera- tively.

The lungs and pulmonary vasculature are protected in patients in whom the shunt flow is from right to left from the outset. Indeed, the pulmonary circulation may fail to develop normally if the flow through it is always small and this sometimes limits the success of surgery, e.g. complete correction of the tetralogy of Fallot. Such patients are always hypoxic but are acclima- tised to a low arterial oxygen tension. They develop secondary polycyth- aemia, and the number of capillaries in some critical vascular beds, e.g. the brain, is increased when cyanosis has been present from birth. The blood is abnormally viscous because of the high haematocrit, tissue perfusion is impaired, and a chronic metabolic acidosis is a common feature (Table 2.2). Disturbances of coagulation mechanisms are sometimes associated with secondary polycythaemia, and both qualitative defects in platelet function

Table 2.2 Results of arterial blood gas analysis on a 3-day-old 3 kg infant suffering from complex cyanotic congenital heart disease. The infant was being nursed in an oxygen-enriched atmosphere, took feeds well and cried lustily when disturbed.

pH	7·34	
PO_2	4·0 kPa	(30 mmHg)
PCO_2	4·0 kPa	(30 mm Hg)
HCO_3	16 mmol/l	

and increased fibrinolytic activity have been reported. Preoperative treatment to correct coagulation abnormalities is sometimes recommended. Paradoxical embolism and cerebral abscess formation are unusual complications of a right to left intracardiac shunt.

Many of the congenital lesions are complex; specific features which are of importance during surgery are discussed individually in Chapters 7 and 9.

EFFECTS OF DRUG THERAPY

Several aspects of cardiac disease are amenable to drug treatment. Digitalis and diuretics are the agents employed most commonly, but anticoagulants, beta-adrenergic blocking drugs, sedatives, hypotensive agents and antibiotics must also be considered.

Digitalis increases the force of contraction of the heart, slows conduction and increases myocardial excitability. It is excreted slowly and can therefore accumulate to reach toxic levels, but dosage is easier to control now that rapid methods are available for assaying plasma digoxin levels; the optimal concentration lies between 1 and 3 ng/ml and values above 4 ng/ml are within the toxic range. Bradycardia or tachydysrhythmias may indicate intoxication, common manifestations being coupled ventricular extrasystoles or paroxysmal atrial tachycardia with block (Fig. 2.2). Digitalis intoxication can be precipitated by hypokalaemia, and latent toxicity may become apparent if the plasma potassium concentration is depressed by the respiratory alkalosis of artificial ventilation. It is customary to discontinue digitalis 36 hours before surgery to minimise the risks of intoxication during the operative period. Even if a measurement of the plasma digoxin concentration is not available, discontinuing therapy preoperatively means that dysrhythmias occurring during surgery are unlikely to be caused by digitalis intoxication and also that the drug can be given, at least in small doses, if a positive indication arises.

Diuretics are prescribed when there is either pulmonary or systemic venous congestion or oedema. Potassium depletion can occur unless

Chapter two

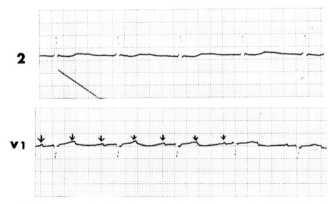

Figure 2.2   Paroxysmal atrial tachycardia with block caused by digitalis intoxication.

supplements are given but may be more closely related to the severity of heart failure than to the adequacy of replacement therapy. Potassium depletion is suggested if the plasma concentration is at or below the lower limit of normal and there is an otherwise unexplained extracellular alkalosis.

When heart failure is particularly severe, prolonged diuretic therapy can deplete the intravascular volume even though there is still an excess of extra-vascular fluid. Hyponatraemia is often present too but does not indicate sodium depletion; it is probably caused by an inability to maintain normal ionic gradients across cell membranes. Hypotension is likely to occur in such patients when vascular tone is reduced by anaesthesia.

Anticoagulants   are used both therapeutically and prophylactically. Patients with a history of systemic embolism may present for surgery when they are fully anticoagulated. Closed procedures, e.g. mitral valvotomy, can be under-taken without the reversal of anticoagulants, and haemorrhage is rarely a problem provided haemostasis is carried out carefully. Anticoagulants are usually withdrawn a few days before open heart surgery (p. 33) but sometimes the prothrombin time fails to return to normal. Vitamin K can be given preoperatively, but more commonly vitamin K and fresh frozen plasma are used postoperatively.

A particular problem occurs when emergency pulmonary embolectomy is required after treatment with streptokinase has already been started. The effects of this fibrinolytic enzyme can be reversed pharmacologically, but in practice it is difficult to determine the optimum dosage of antifibrinolytic drugs and often wiser to rely on transfusion with fresh frozen plasma or fresh whole blood (p. 129).

Beta-adrenergic blocking agents are given to control some tachydys-rhythmias, to relieve anginal pain, and to decrease ventricular outflow tract obstruction in conditions such as the tetralogy of Fallot or hypertrophic obstructive cardiomyopathy. These drugs are all myocardial depressants although some separation of the negative inotropic and chronotropic effects has been achieved with the newer representatives.

Anaesthesia and cardiac surgery always entail some myocardial depression. Intractable heart failure can result if the heart is already depressed by beta-adrenergic blocking agents, and the usual supportive drugs are likely to prove ineffective. Large doses of beta-adrenergic stimulants (e.g. isoprenaline) produce slight improvement in myocardial function, but drugs with both alpha- and beta-adrenergic stimulant properties (e.g. adrenaline) merely increase the peripheral resistance whilst the effect on contractility is minimal. Glucagon (p. 95) remains effective. It has been argued that beta-adrenergic blocking agents should be withdrawn preoperatively for anything from 2 days to 2 weeks. However, recent reports have emphasised that symptoms and sequelae of ischaemic heart disease can be exacerbated by the withdrawal of propranolol or its derivatives and there is a growing tendency to continue beta-adrenergic blockade up to the time of surgery.

Hypotensive drugs are taken occasionally by patients who are being prepared for cardiac surgery, either because they suffer from coexistent hypertension or because antihypertensive therapy has been prescribed specifically for the cardiac lesion, for example, acute dissection of the aorta. In both circumstances, it is probably less hazardous to continue the drug than to withdraw it long enough before operation for the effects to wear off. It is necessary to control the blood volume with particular care during surgery, and to use circulatory stimulants with caution because several antihypertensive agents increase the sensitivity of autonomic receptors to adrenergic stimuli.

Sedatives are often prescribed for the anxiety which so commonly accompanies cardiac disease. Some patients are given antidepressants and monoamine oxidase inhibitors are chosen occasionally. The latter have also been used in the past to control anginal pain and to treat hypertension. They compromise both anaesthetic management and circulatory support and must be discontinued at least 3 weeks before cardiac surgery.

Other drugs used in the management of cardiac disease include coronary vasodilators, antibiotics, and agents designed to lower elevated levels of serum cholesterol and triglycerides; none have any particular significance for the anaesthetist. Diabetic partients presenting for cardiac surgery are handled in the usual way. It is important to note that the blood sugar is generally elevated after cardiopulmonary bypass in normal subjects, particularly if large volumes of solutions containing glucose have been used to prime the oxygenator or if hypothermia has been employed.

Patients requiring essential drugs not listed here (e.g. anticonvulsants) should have their usual regime restarted as soon as possible after operation. Parenteral administration is necessary if the gastrointestinal route is impractical.

REFERENCES

PULMONARY SEQUELAE OF CARDIAC DISEASE

ABERMAN A. & FULOP M. (1972) The metabolic and respiratory acidosis of acute pulmonary oedema. *Annals of Internal Medicine* **76**, 173.

AVERY W. G., SAMET P. & SACKNER M.A. (1970) The acidosis of pulmonary edema. *American Journal of Medicine* **48**, 320.

BASS H. (1972) Emphysema and mitral valve disease. *Chest* **62**, 9.

FRIEDBERG C. K. (1971) Oedema and pulmonary oedema: pathologic physiology and differential diagnosis. *Progress in Cardiovascular Diseases* **13**, 546.

LANGE R. K. & HECHT H. H. (1962) The mechanism of Cheyne-Stokes respiration. *Journal of Clinical Investigation* **41**, 42.

LAVER M. B., HALLOWELL P. & GOLDBLATT A. (1970) Pulmonary dysfunction secondary to heart disease: aspects relevant to anesthesia and surgery. *Anesthesiology* **33**, 161.

SCHREINER B. F. Jr., MURPHY G. W., KRAMER D. H., SHAH P. M., MARX H. J. & YU P. N. (1971) Pathophysiology of pulmonary congestion. *Progress in Cardiovascular Diseases* **14**, 57.

ZELIS R., NELLIS S. H., LONGHURST J., LEE G. & MASON D. T. (1975) Abnormalities in the regional circulations accompanying congestive heart failure. *Progress in Cardiovascular Diseases* **18**, 181.

DYSRHYTHMIAS

KATZ R. L. & BIGGER J. T. (1970) Cardiac arrhythmias during anesthesia and operation. *Anesthesiology* **33**, 193.

SCHAMROTH L. (1971) *An Introduction to Electrocardiography*, 4th Ed. Blackwell Scientific Publications, Oxford.

SOME CONSEQUENCES OF CONGENITAL HEART DISEASE

EKERT H. & SHEERS M. (1974). Pre-operative and post-operative platelet function in cyanotic congenital heart disease. *Journal of Thoracic and Cardiovascular Surgery* **67**, 184.

GRALNICK H. R. (1970). Epsilon-aminocaproic acid in pre-operative correction of haemostatic defect in cyanotic congenital heart disease. *Lancet* **1**, 1204.

HALLIDIE-SMITH K. A. & GOODWIN J. F. (1974) The Eisenmenger syndrome. In *Progress in Cardiology* Ed. P. N. Yu & J. F. Goodwin, p. 211. Lea & Febiger, Philadelphia.

KOMP, D. M. & SPARROW, A. W. (1970) Polycythaemia in cyanotic heart disease: a study of altered coagulation. *Journal of Pediatrics* **76**, 231.

STOELTING R. K. & LONGNECKER D. W. (1972) The effect of right to left shunt on the rate of increase of arterial anesthetic concentration. *Anesthesiology* **36**, 352.

DRUG THERAPY

Digitalis

Leading Article (1975) Problems with digoxin. *British Medical Journal* **1**, 49.

Diuretics/Electrolyte Disturbances

DONALDSON E. K., PATRICK J., SIVAPRAGASM S., WOO MING M. O. & ALLEYNE G. A. O. (1976) Effect of triamterene on leucocyte sodium and potassium levels in heart disease. *British Medical Journal* **2**, 1254.

EDMONSON R. P. S., THOMAS R. D., HILTON P. J., PATRICK J. & JONES N. F. (1974) Leucocyte electrolytes in cardiac and non-cardiac patients receiving diuretics. *Lancet* **1**, 12.

HOLDEN M. P., IONESCU M. I. & WOOLER G. H. (1971) Magnesium in patients undergoing open-heart surgery. *Thorax* **27**, 212.

Leading Article (1975) Calcium, magnesium, and diuretics. *British Medical Journal* **1**, 170.

SELLER R. H. (1971) The role of magnesium in digitalis toxicity. *American Heart Journal* **82**, 551.

VAUGHAN R. S. & LUNN J. N. (1973) Potassium and the anaesthetist: a review. *Anaesthesia* **28**, 118.

WHITE R. J. (1970) Effect of potassium supplements on the exchangeable potassium in chronic heart disease. *British Medical Journal* **3**, 141.

Anticoagulants

ELLISON N. & OMINSKY A. J. (1973) Clinical considerations for the anesthesiologist whose patient is on anticoagulant therapy. *Anesthesiology* **39**, 328.

Beta-adrenergic blocking drugs

ALDERMAN E. L., COLTART D. J., WETTACH G. E. & HARRISON D. C. (1974) Coronary artery syndromes after sudden propranolol withdrawal. *Annals of Internal Medicine* **81**, 625.

FAULKNER S. L., HOPKINS J. T. & BOERTH R. C. (1973) Time required for complete recovery from chronic propranolol therapy. *New England Journal of Medicine* **289**, 607.

HARRISON D. C. & ALDERMAN E. L. (1976) Discontinuation of propranolol therapy. Cause of rebound angina pectoris and acute coronary events. *Chest* **69**, 1.

KAPLAN J. A., DUNBAR R. W., BLAND J. W. Jr., SUMPTER R. & JONES E. L. (1975) Propranolol and cardiac surgery: a problem for the anesthesiologist? *Current Researches in Anesthesia and Analgesia* **54**, 571.

SHAND D. G. (1975) Propranolol withdrawal. *New England Journal of Medicine* **292**, 449.

VILJOEN J. F., ESTAFANOUS G. & KELLNER G. A. (1972) Propranolol and cardiac surgery. *Journal of Thoracic and Cardiovascular Surgery* **64**, 826.

Hypotensive drug therapy

HICKLER R. B. & VANDAM D. (1970) Hypertension. *Anesthesiology* **33**, 214.

FOEX P. & PRYS-ROBERTS C. (1974) Anaesthesia and the hypertensive patient. *British Journal of Anaesthesia* **46**, 575.

CHAPTER 3

PREOPERATIVE ASSESSMENT AND PREPARATION

The information required by the anaesthetist about a patient presenting for cardiac surgery can be listed as follows:

1 What is the cardiac lesion and what form of surgery is proposed?
2 What sequelae have resulted in the individual patient and how rapidly is the condition changing?
3 Are there any other features of importance, not necessarily related to cardiac disease?
4 Has optimal preoperative preparation been achieved?

Answers to these questions are obtained at a preoperative visit which also provides an opportunity for meeting the patient, assessing his physique and personality, and establishing rapport.

CARDIOLOGICAL DIAGNOSIS

The nature of the cardiac lesion is sometimes apparent on routine clinical examination, corroborated by a chest X-ray and ECG. Other investigations are required if the diagnosis is in doubt, or if more precise information is required to evaluate whether surgery is desirable or even feasible. Such studies include cardiac catheterisation, angiography and echocardiography. Some of the specialised aspects of their interpretation are of little practical significance to the anaesthetist but they may also reveal information which is invaluable, for example, an angiographic assessment of left ventricular contractility, a measurement of cardiac output at rest, a calculated value for pulmonary vascular resistance and measurements of arterial oxygen content or saturation.

Although one or more of these investigations will have been carried out on most patients, it is important to appreciate that they are not done routinely. Straightforward cases are often submitted for surgery with nothing more elaborate than a chest X-ray and ECG, together with some simple biochemical and haematological tests (pp. 30 and 31).

The nature of the operation governs posture during surgery and the choice of anaesthetic and monitoring techniques (Chapters 5 and 6). Knowledge of the procedure also permits some prediction of the magnitude of the operative risks and the nature and likelihood of complications.

ASSESSMENT OF THE INDIVIDUAL PATIENT

The evaluation of sequelae within an individual patient is partly a matter of knowing what to expect. A general account of the effects of cardiac disease is given in Chapter 2 and important aspects of particular conditions are discussed in Chapters 5 and 7.

History and examination

A detailed history is often available in the casenotes but it is worth taking it again, at least in broad outline, because the conversation provides an opportunity for appreciating the patient's reaction to his disease as well as the relative importance of different symptoms. Questions are aimed at eliciting the extent of functional impairment and certain specific points should be covered:

Is the patient's exercise tolerance impaired? If so, to what extent and how consistently? Is the limiting factor breathlessness, pain, or fatigue? If pain, what is its nature and does it also occur at rest? If dyspnoea is a troublesome feature, is it variable? paroxysmal? nocturnal? Is the patient wheezy? Does he have any cough? produce any phlegm? take any regular medication for his breathing? What are his smoking habits? Is he abnormally prone to respiratory tract infections? Answers to these questions provide information about both cardiac and pulmonary disability and may indicate the need for further investigation.

Rhythm disturbances often pass unnoticed by the patient although he may admit to palpitations, especially if the sensation is described to him in simple terms. It is important to elicit this history because dysrhythmias are a common cause of circulatory disturbances during and after surgery. Observant patients can tell whether the heart beat is regular or irregular, how the attack starts and stops, whether or not he feels faint or cold, and whether he has been noticed to change colour or sweat.

Syncope may result from rhythm changes but transitory episodes of loss of consciousness can also be caused by an abrupt decrease in cardiac output without rhythm change (e.g. effort syncope in aortic stenosis, cyanotic attacks in Fallot's tetralogy). Cerebral embolism is another cause of slightly more prolonged periods of altered consciousness, often accompanied by disturbances of speech or vision. Alternatively systemic embolism can cause symptoms of transitory ischaemia in a limb.

The totally non-specific question 'What is your general health like?' sometimes elicits replies which are unexpectedly revealing. Gastrointestinal disturbances, urinary tract infections, intermittent claudication and symptoms related to cerebrovascular disease may be mentioned, together with a great deal of largely irrelevant information. Some of these symptoms may be important, particularly those suggestive of cerebrovascular disease, because such patients are often unable to tolerate the hypotension and haemodilution of extracorporeal circulation and show an increased incidence of postoperative neurological damage.

Questions about 'general health' can be followed by a few more specific points such as past medical history, details of previous anaesthetic experience, any allergies or drug idiosyncrasies and an account of current medication. Drugs prescribed for the cardiac condition may have been noted already, but the question is worth asking because so many patients also take regular therapy for unrelated disorders. Finally, enquiry should be made into the state of the teeth. Whether or not the patient has received recent dental treatment and whether or not this was covered with antibiotic therapy may be important information in patients admitted with suspected subacute bacterial endocarditis, but the anaesthetist is much more concerned with the present dental state and whether or not his manœuvres at the time of surgery will liberate showers of organisms into the circulation.

The physical examination is directed towards an evaluation of the functional state of the various systems rather than to the finer points of cardiological diagnosis. Is there evidence of pulmonary or systemic venous congestion? Is the peripheral circulation well perfused? Are there signs of pulmonary disease, either as a feature of the cardiac lesion or as an unrelated abnormality? Is the patient obese or abnormally wasted? Is he cyanosed or jaundiced? Are there any anatomical features of practical anaesthetic significance such as prominent or loose teeth or a small jaw? Are the peripheral pulses present and symmetrical? A pulse may be absent because of previous embolism or cannulation but sometimes an exaggerated pulse is palpable distal to the site of cardiac catheterisation, possibly indicating vasodilatation following minor damage to the autonomic nerve fibres carried on the surface of the vessel.

While the history is being taken and the patient examined, the rate of progression of his disease can be assessed in the context of the natural history of the particular condition. Rapid deterioration is important because it restricts both the time available for lengthy preoperative preparation and the development of compensatory mechanisms by the patient. This in turn influences the interpretation of abnormal findings. For example, a left atrial pressure of 25 mm Hg (3·3 kPa) or more will cause pulmonary oedema in patients with previously normal lungs, whereas those with a chronically elevated left atrial pressure develop pulmonary vascular changes (Chapter 2) which enable them to tolerate much higher pressures without further acute deterioration.

Chest X-ray and ECG

Physical examination is followed by consideration of the ECG and chest X-ray. Postero-anterior and lateral films are taken routinely and reveal the size and shape of the heart, atria and great vessels, the degree of vascularisation of the lung fields, and the presence of intracardiac or pericardial calcification. An overpenetrated P–A view may be required to confirm left atrial enlargement and often demonstrates calcification more clearly. Intracardiac (valvar) calcification is common on the left side of the heart, particularly on the aortic valve; calcification around the heart is relatively uncommon and signifies pericardial disease but not necessarily constriction of cardiac chambers.

The state of the pulmonary vasculature is assessed by noting the size of the pulmonary arteries and the degree of vascularisation of the peripheral

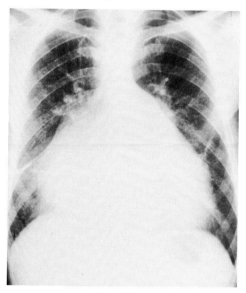

Figure 3.1 Chest X-ray of a 42-year-old male with severe mitral valve disease. There is cardiomegaly, dilatation of the upper lobe veins and pleural fluid in the lesser fissure; septal lines are visible in the lower zones.

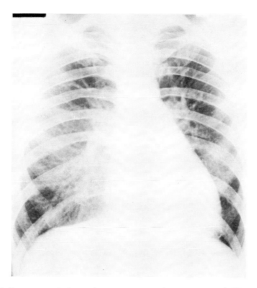

Figure 3.2 Pulmonary plethora in a symptom-free man aged 33 years who was shown to have a secundum type atrial septal defect.

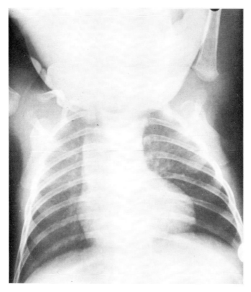

Figure 3.3 'Macrogram' (magnified chest X-ray) of an 8-month-old child with cyanotic heart disease (tetralogy of Fallot) and pulmonary oligaemia.

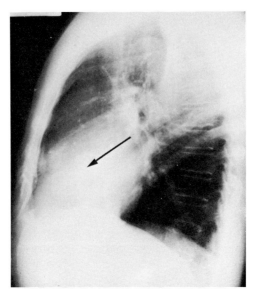

Figure 3.4   Lateral chest X-ray showing calcification of the aortic valve in a man
of 70 with aortic stenosis who presented with syncopal attacks.

lung fields; pulmonary venous hypertension is indicated by upper lobe blood
diversion and lymphatic obstruction (Kerley B lines).

There may be abnormalities in the lung fields or pleural cavities. Small
pleural effusions are common in heart failure and there is occasionally partial
or complete collapse of the left lower lobe caused by pressure of an enlarged
left atrium on the lower lobe bronchus.

The ECG should be inspected for evidence of rhythm disturbances, ventricular hypertrophy, strain or myocardial ischaemia.

Laboratory investigations

The need for specialised cardiodiagnostic techniques has been discussed previously (p. 25); other investigations which may be required are detailed
below.

Haematology   A full blood count is requested and should include red cell
indices and inspection of a stained film; a platelet count is not always carried
out unless the smear suggests they are deficient in numbers or there is a history
of abnormal bleeding. The prothrombin time is measured in patients receiving anticoagulants and should be repeated a day or two later if these drugs
are discontinued (p. 33). Other coagulation studies may be indicated in special
circumstances, for example, cyanotic congenital heart disease with secondary
polycythaemia (p. 18).

Four to eight units of blood are cross-matched for surgery on adult patients. This should be as fresh as possible, especially if required for cardio-pulmonary bypass, and fresh heparinised blood is sometimes collected on the morning of operation. All donors as well as the recipient should be screened for Australia antigen.

Biochemistry A routine urine test is carried out on the ward. Slight pro-teinuria is common in heart failure and some patients using thiazide diuretics develop hyperglycaemia and glycosuria. Heavy proteinuria or haematuria suggest that further investigation of the renal tract is necessary.

The plasma electrolytes and urea are always determined and abnormal values are commonly detected. Elevation of the blood urea may be a mani-festation of heart failure, overzealous diuretic therapy or of renal disease. Hypokalaemia is often caused by diuretic therapy (p. 19) and total body potassium depletion is usually associated with an extracellular alkalosis. Most laboratories quote a value for at least one plasma anion (either chloride or bicarbonate) and it is generally possible to deduce from this whether or not an alkalosis is present. There is then no need to request more detailed assessment by analysis of arterial blood unless there is some additional reason for pH and blood gas measurements (p. 32).

Hyponatraemia, another common finding in patients with severe cardiac disease who have been treated with diuretics, is sometimes present when there is still peripheral oedema, i.e. a manifest excess of extracellular sodium (p. 20). The low sodium concentration cannot be corrected by the administration of hypertonic sodium solutions and attempts to do so are generally disastrous.

Renal function should be assessed in greater detail if the elevation of blood urea is disproportionate to other manifestations of the patient's disease, or if analysis of the urine suggests that renal function is abnormal. Liver function tests are indicated in patients who are jaundiced, in those who have tricuspid valve disease and those who have suffered from prolonged systemic venous congestion.

Bacteriology A nasal swab is collected on admission to hospital, but other cultures (e.g. skin, sputum, urine) are only set up when indicated. 'Naseptin' cream and 'Phisohex' baths are often prescribed to minimise carriage of strains of *Staphylococcus aureus*.

Assessment of pulmonary function

Dyspnoea and derangements of pulmonary function are common in patients with cardiac disease, but detailed studies are rarely undertaken unless the respiratory disability is both chronic and severe, or there is evidence of signifi-cant but unrelated pulmonary disease. In such cases, a reasonable minimum is spirometry to determine the ratio of forced expiratory volume in one second to forced vital capacity (FEV_1/FVC), and to observe the effect on it of bronchodilator drugs. Measurements of total lung capacity and its subdivisions, or of the transfer factor are interesting but rarely of practical importance, and are sometimes difficult to interpret in the presence of both cardiac and pulmonary pathology (p. 12). Arterial blood gas analysis may be indicated to detect hypercapnia in patients with severe airways obstruction, and it is sometimes helpful to know the extent of arterial hypoxaemia. Analysis of arterial blood is particularly useful prior to emergency surgery because it enables the degree of metabolic acidosis to be assessed accurately in patients with circulatory failure.

PREOPERATIVE PREPARATION

The time devoted to preoperative preparation depends on the degree of functional disturbance and the likelihood of achieving improvement by medical means; there is no time for any preoperative preparation in patients with immediately life-threatening circulatory failure.

Those with stable cardiac disease without heart failure require only a day or two in hospital before surgery. This provides time for essential investigations to be completed and an opportunity for preoperative physiotherapy. The patient's informed cooperation will be needed in the postoperative period, and he and his relatives must be told what to expect in the way of transfer to an Intensive Care Unit, chest drains, the endotracheal tube and artificial ventilation. Breathing exercises, assisted coughing, and, possibly, the use of intermittent positive pressure breathing are all explained and practised, and the necessity for continuing these manœuvres postoperatively is emphasised.

Patients with clinical signs of heart failure benefit from a longer period of preparation. Bed rest, oxygen therapy if necessary, and optimal doses of digitalis and diuretics will often eliminate signs of heart failure. The cardiac rate and rhythm are controlled as far as possible although it is sometimes considered undesirable to use beta-adrenergic blocking agents preoperatively (p. 21). If possible, surgery is delayed in patients with subacute bacterial endocarditis or active rheumatic carditis until the disease is controlled or quiescent. Similarly, it is preferable to delay operation for at least 3 months in patients with a completed myocardial infarct. Those with ischaemic heart disease suffering from crescendo angina, recurrent rhythm disturbances, or intractable heart failure related to a ruptured ventricular septum, chordal rupture or large left ventricular aneurysm may however require operation as an emergency.

Patients with pulmonary disease should be encouraged to stop smoking, even if only for a relatively short time. Oral or respiratory tract infection should be treated and bronchodilator therapy may be needed. Salbutamol, 2·5–5·0 mg delivered three or four times a day by intermittent positive pressure breathing from a 'Bird' nebuliser, is an effective bronchodilator and unlikely to cause any disturbance of cardiac rhythm. The treatment can be accompanied by postural drainage if the cardiac condition permits, or by assisted coughing only.

Anaemia should be corrected if possible, but a transfusion of stored blood given the day before operation probably does more harm than good. In some centres, blood is collected from the patient preoperatively and stored for replacement at the time of surgery; preoperative anaemia is an accepted feature of this technique.

The optimum management of patients receiving long-term anticoagulant treatment is difficult to define. There is a definite risk of thrombosis when anticoagulants are withdrawn, particularly if the prothrombin time is corrected quickly with vitamin K. On the other hand, it is important to ensure that iatrogenic coagulation disturbances do not interfere with the control of blood loss at operation. The risks of haemorrhage during surgery in patients receiving coumarin-type anticoagulants are slight provided haemostasis is meticulous, and closed cardiac surgery is often undertaken on fully anticoagulated patients with a prothrombin ratio of 2 : 1. Haemorrhage is a much greater hazard during open heart surgery. Anticoagulants are generally withdrawn a day or two beforehand although few surgeons insist on a normal prothrombin time preoperatively and are content to rely on the transfusion of coagulation factors in blood and plasma given during the operation.

Digitalis and diuretics are generally discontinued 36 hours preoperatively. This rarely leads to any loss of control of heart failure but decreases the risks of drug-induced dysrhythmias during the biochemical derangements which so often accompany anaesthesia, controlled ventilation and cardiopulmonary bypass (pp. 19, 83).

PREMEDICATION

It is sometimes argued that sympathetic preoperative visit and the use of non-irritant anaesthetic techniques eliminate the need for premedication with all its attendant side-effects. Although a sympathetic preoperative visit is always helpful, it is rarely sufficient to quell the anxiety which accompanies major surgery for heart disease. Anxiety is detrimental to morale and causes a tachycardia which is also undesirable. Similarly, salivation, bronchorrhoea and rhythm changes induced by stimulation of the respiratory tract are potentially hazardous and cannot always be avoided, no matter how careful the technique. In some circumstances, generous sedation is a positive advantage. It permits the use of smaller doses of anaesthetic agents which are themselves depressant. In patients with pulmonary oedema and good left ventricular function, it decreases hyperventilation with its consequent hypocapnia and vasoconstriction, decreases left ventricular work by lowering the systemic vascular resistance, and decreases pulmonary engorgement by dilating the systemic capacitance vessels. Finally, in those with the tetralogy of Fallot, sedation with opiates prevents or alleviates spasm of the outflow tract of the right ventricle (p. 122).

Hyperventilation is common in many forms of cardiac disease and consequently there is less risk than usual of causing respiratory depression with excessive doses of preoperative sedatives. The duration of most operations is such that postoperative respiratory depression cannot be attributed to premedication, while in many cases artificial ventilation is continued postoperatively for other reasons. As a general rule, therefore, sedative premedication should be generous. Hyoscine is preferable to atropine as a vagolytic because it provides additional sedation and is much less likely to cause an undesirable tachycardia.

Many patients appreciate a hypnotic the night before operation. The following day, premedication is given 1 hour before leaving the ward. Papaveretum (10–20 mg) with hyoscine (0·2–0·4 mg) is a satisfactory combination for most adults; a barbiturate, neuroleptic agent or benzodiazepine can be added for robust patients. Ideally, the patient is conscious but tranquil on arrival in the anaesthetic room. Generous sedative premedication is particularly necessary for young patients with mitral stenosis (p. 57), those with ischaemic heart disease (p. 116), and those with the tetralogy of Fallot (p. 122).

Heavy premedication should be avoided in certain cases. Patients requiring emergency cardiac surgery generally do not need any sedation and are best managed with a small dose of hyoscine or atropine, the risks of tachycardia with the latter being unimportant when the heart rate is already very high. Patients with severe pulmonary disease complicating long-standing pulmonary hypertension cannot be sedated heavily for fear of respiratory depression, while those with a low cardiac output who are critically dependent on an adequate filling pressure (aortic stenosis, cardiac tamponade or constrictive pericarditis) should be sedated with caution. Patients with tight aortic stenosis and signs of circulatory failure are particularly vulnerable to vasodilating drugs because the reduction in filling pressure is accompanied by a decrease in arteriolar tone; the lowered arterial pressure which results may be inadequate to perfuse the hypertrophied left ventricle.

Patients with severe, long-standing heart failure are often cachectic and sometimes jaundiced or uraemic. Reduced doses of premedicant drugs should be given in these circumstances. Anxious patients in whom for one reason or another opiates are considered to be contraindicated can often be sedated safely with a small dose of diazepam (2·5–7·5 mg). This is given intramuscularly or by mouth, accompanied by the usual dose of hyoscine, and the combination produces very little depression of either respiration or circulation.

REFERENCES

FLEMING P. R. (1974) Cardiological aspects of the pre-operative examination. *British Journal of Anaesthesia* **46,** 555.

GOLDSTEIN A. & KEATS A. S. (1970) The risk of anaesthesia. *Anesthesiology* **33,** 130.

HAMER J. (1976) Today's treatment—cardiac failure. *British Medical Journal* **3,** 220.

KERR I. H. (1974) The pre-operative chest X-ray. *British Journal of Anaesthesia* **46,** 558.

LYONS S. M., CLARKE R. S. J., VULGARAKI K. (1975) Premedication of cardiac surgical patients: a clinical comparison of four regimes. *Anaesthesia* **30,** 459.

For references on preoperative drug therapy, see Chapter 2.

ANAESTHESIA FOR DIAGNOSTIC PROCEDURES

Successful cardiac surgery can only be undertaken if both the anatomy and the functional state of the heart are clearly appreciated. It is often impossible to obtain this information by clinical examination, and additional investigation may be required using methods which are described in this chapter.

CARDIAC CATHETERISATION AND ANGIOCARDIOGRAPHY

Right heart catheterisation is usually carried out from an antecubital or brachial vein which is exposed surgically; the axillary or femoral veins are sometimes chosen in small infants. The tip of the catheter can virtually always be guided under radiological control into the great veins, the right atrium, right ventricle and pulmonary artery, and the left heart can be entered too if there is either a patent foramen ovale or an abnormal communication between the two sides of the heart. In most cases, the catheter can be advanced through the pulmonary arterial system until it impacts in a vessel of comparable diameter; pressure recorded from this site, the 'pulmonary arterial wedge pressure', is a good indication of pressure in the left atrium, provided a fairly small catheter (e.g. OD 2·0–2·5 mm) without multiple side-holes is used.

Interpretation of the wedge pressure can be difficult, particularly if there is pulmonary vascular disease, and it is sometimes necessary to enter the left atrium directly. Transeptal puncture can be carried out by advancing a long needle, protected by an outer catheter, from the femoral vein into the right atrium. The tip is manipulated until it lodges in the foramen ovale, and the needle is then pushed on through the septum into the left atrium. The catheter can then be advanced into the left ventricle. This chamber is approached more commonly by retrograde catheterisation from either the brachial or femoral artery, and retrograde catheterisation is also the usual approach for investigating the coronary arterial system.

When the brachial artery is used, the vessel is exposed at the same time as the vein. The catheter is introduced through a small arteriotomy which is repaired when the procedure has been completed. Cannulation of the femoral artery is often performed percutaneously using the Seldinger technique. A flexible guide wire is introduced through a short needle in the artery; the needle is then withdrawn and the catheter is threaded over the wire and on into the artery. Unless the arteries are tortuous or atheromatous, it is usually easy to pass the catheter into the ascending aorta. It is then manipulated so that the tip passes through the aortic valve into the left ventricle, or enters the coronary arteries. It is also possible to enter the left atrium by this route.

Cardiac catheterisation is usually accompanied by angiocardiography. Radioopaque contrast medium is injected under pressure, and its passage through the heart is recorded either on serial films exposed in quick succession, or by cineradiography. Biplane recording (two films exposed in planes at right angles to each other) is used to provide a three-dimensional image of the heart. If contrast medium is injected through a wide-bore catheter with a single end-hole, the tip may recoil violently when the injection is made, so depositing the injectate in an unwanted site. This problem is eliminated if the catheter is changed before the angiogram for one with multiple sideholes proximal to an occluded tip.

Measurement and interpretation of intracardiac pressures

Dynamic and mean pressures can be recorded from the chambers and vessels reached by the catheter but satisfactory measurements can only be made through a hydrostatic system which has an adequate frequency response. The minimum requirement is twenty cycles per second but the performance of modern apparatus is vastly better than this; provided non-distensible tubing is used and the system is free from trapped bubbles.

The catheters and transducers are sterilised before use and flushed to remove irritant substances. Once the catheter has been inserted, it should be flushed periodically with heparinised saline or Ringer-lactate solution to prevent blood entering the tip. Heparin (5–10 000 units) is sometimes given before arterial catheterisation to prevent thrombosis at the arteriotomy site or the formation of clot on the outer wall of the catheter which could be swept off when the catheter is withdrawn.

An important consideration is the zero point to which all pressures are referred. During clinical examination, it is customary to judge the height of the venous pressure against the sternal angle but this is not the ideal reference point for structures which are situated more posteriorly, in particular the left atrium. Alternative reference points in common use are the mid-axillary line or, in adult patients, 10 cm in front of the vertebral column.

Table 4.1   Normal values for pressures in the heart and great vessels referred to zero at the mid-axillary line. From Yang *et al.*, 1972.

	Range (mm Hg)	Average (mm Hg)	(kPa)
Mean right atrium	1–5	2·8	0·4
Right ventricle			
systolic	17–32	25	3·3
end-diastolic	1– 7	4	0·5
Pulmonary artery			
systolic	17–32	25	3·3
end-diastolic	4–13	9	1·2
mean	9–19	15	2·0
Pulmonary arterial			
'wedge'	4·5–13	9	1·2
Mean left atrium	2–12	7·9	1·1
Left ventricle			
systolic	90–140	130	17·3
end-diastolic	5–12	8·7	1·2
Systemic artery			
systolic	90–140	130	17·3
diastolic	60–90	70	9.3
mean	70–105	85	11·3

Although the difference between these levels is fairly small for a supine, horizontal subject and may be of little significance when dealing with pressure in the systemic arteries or left ventricle, serious confusion can be introduced when atrial or pulmonary arterial pressures are being discussed. Normal values for intracardiac pressures referred to zero at the mid-axillary line are quoted in Table 4.1.

The units of measurement can also be a source of misunderstanding. The venous pressure judged clinically is usually expressed as cm of water (or saline or blood) but intracardiac pressures are generally quoted in mm Hg. The numerical discrepancy between these units is fairly small when low pressures are being considered (13.6 cm $H_2O = 10$ mm Hg) but becomes of greater importance at higher levels of pressure. A final difficulty has been introduced in the recent past by the advent of SI units. Although widely accepted for

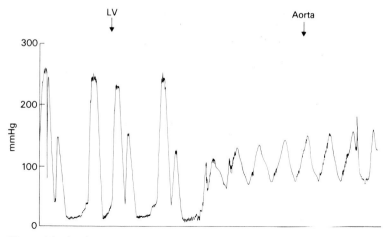

Figure 4.1 Aortic stenosis: male aged 68. Withdrawal trace across the aortic valve—extrasystoles account for the irregularity of successive beats. The right heart pressures were normal but the 'wedge' pressure was elevated: Mean right atrium: 2 mm Hg (0·3 kPa); Right ventricle: 32/2 mm Hg (4·3/0·3 kPa); Mean pulmonary arterial 'wedge': 18 mm Hg (2·4 kPa); Cardiac index: 2·0 l min^{-1} m^{-2}.

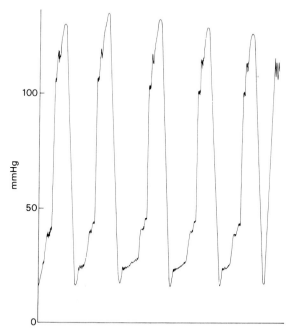

Figure 4.2 Ischaemic heart disease: male aged 42. Gross elevation of the left ventricular end-diastolic pressure in the absence of valvular disease.

expressing the chemical composition of blood and body fluids, there has been great reluctance to employ the kilopascal for the expression of haemodynamic pressures. Throughout this text, pressure measurements have been expressed in mm Hg with the corresponding value in kPa in brackets.

Abnormal elevation of intracardiac pressures can arise in a number of ways. There may be distal obstruction caused by a stenosed valve (Fig. 4.1), or by vasoconstriction or obliteration of a vascular bed; functional stenosis can result from the passage of a very high flow through an orifice of normal size.

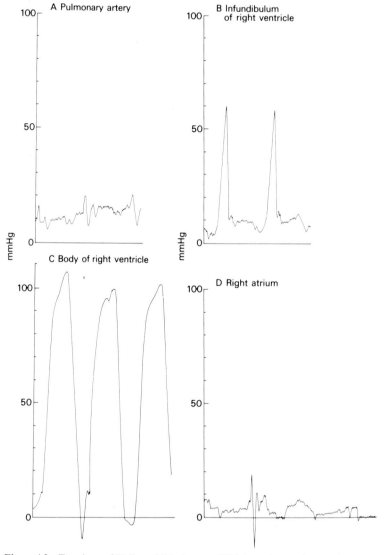

Figure 4.3 Tetralogy of Fallot: child, 4 years. Withdrawal trace from pulmonary artery, through right ventricle to right atrium. The ratio of pulmonary to systemic blood flow (Q_p/Q_s) was 0·8 and the child showed slight arterial desaturation at rest (92%).

Elevated pressures will also be detected if there is an abnormal communication between two chambers of different pressure (e.g. valvular regurgitation or some intracardiac shunts), and passive transmission of pressure in a retrograde direction may be detected as abnormal elevation in a more proximal site, e.g. pulmonary arterial hypertension secondary to the raised left atrial pressure of early mitral stenosis. Finally, intracardiac pressures can be elevated when the gross anatomy of the heart is normal but functional impairment has resulted in an increase in both the end-diastolic fibre length and the distending pressure within the heart (Fig. 4.2).

Pulmonary arterial hypertension is of particular importance and the causes are listed below:

1 Passive (Pulmonary vascular resistance (PVR) normal)
   (i) retrograde transmission of pressure from pulmonary veins or left atrium, e.g. mitral valve disease.
   (ii) abnormally high pulmonary blood flow, e.g. atrial septal defect.

2 Active (PVR elevated)
   (i) pulmonary arteriolar constriction, e.g. in response to the high flow and pressure caused by an uncomplicated ventricular septal defect. PVR elevated but reversible.
   (ii) pulmonary vascular obliteration, e.g. endarteritis, thromboembolism, emphysema. PVR elevated and fixed.

The significance of elevated pressures can only be appreciated fully if the flow rate of blood at that site is known too. This is particularly true when

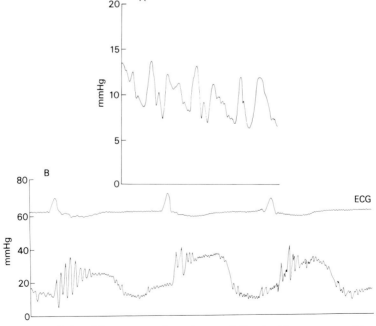

Figure 4.4 Left atrial pressure tracings: A, normal; B, mitral incompetence. (Note the different scales.)

the pressure gradient across a stenosed orifice is being evaluated because the gradient may be trivial in spite of severe stenosis if forward flow is very small.

Abnormally low pressures are seen much less commonly but may be detected distal to an obstruction, or if there is an unusually low flow through the chamber in question. A good example is the pulmonary arterial hypotension which occurs in patients with the tetralogy of Fallot, where there is both a low flow through the pulmonary artery and proximal stenosis at the level of the right ventricular outflow tract (Fig. 4.3).

Information can sometimes be obtained from the contours of the dynamic waveform, for example the dominant 'v' wave which is seen in the left atrial pressure trace when the mitral valve is incompetent (Fig. 4.4). Changes in the waveform may provide sufficient information to establish the diagnosis, but in general do not indicate the magnitude of the defect.

Significance of measurements of oxygen saturation

The oxygen saturation of blood samples withdrawn from various sites in the heart and great vessels is usually determined by oximetry. Oxygen content can then be calculated if the haemoglobin or oxygen-carrying capacity of the blood are known, or alternatively, oxygen content can be measured directly.

An unexpected change in oxygen saturation between samples withdrawn

Table 4.2. Ventricular septal defect: child aged 2 years. Oxygen saturation at various sites within the heart and great veins. The left and right ventricular pressures were 85/12 mm Hg (11·3/1·6 kPa) and 70/5 mm Hg (9·3/0·7 kPa) respectively, and the ratio of pulmonary to systemic blood flow (Q_p/Q_s) was 1.9.

	satn. %
High superior vena cava	73
High right atrium	55
Mid-right atrium	58
Low right atrium	65
High inferior vena cava	72
Low inferior vena cava	76
Right ventricular outflow tract	94
Right pulmonary artery	84
Left atrium	99
Left ventricular apex	99

Table 4.3 Maximum normal variation in oxygen content between adjacent sites reached during right heart catheterisation. From Yang *et al.*, 1972.

	Maximum increase in oxygen content over proximal chamber (vol %)
Pulmonary artery	0.5
Right ventricle	0·9
Right atrium	1·9

from adjacent chambers suggests mixing with blood originating from a different site, for example, a sudden increase in saturation between right atrial and right ventricular samples indicates the presence of a left to right shunt through a ventricular septal defect (Table 4.2). The maximum normal variation in oxygen saturation between adjacent chambers is given in Table 4.3. These differences are caused by streaming of blood in the chambers of the heart, or by the entry of blood through the coronary sinus and other vessels.

Estimations of flow can be made on the basis of the Fick principle if the oxygen content of both arterial and venous blood and the subject's oxygen consumption are known. Basal values for oxygen consumption are often assumed but it is preferable to measure oxygen uptake individually by analysing expired gas collected at the same time as the blood samples. If there is an intracardiac shunt, blood flow through the lungs and the systemic circulation is not necessarily the same, and pulmonary arterial samples may not be representative of mixed systemic venous blood. When this problem arises, the systemic venous oxygen saturation is usually derived by assuming that blood in the inferior and superior venae cavae contributes in a fixed proportion: a formula which provides good correlation with true mixed venous blood is $(3SVC + high IVC) \times \frac{1}{4}$. Systemic blood flow can then be determined by dividing oxygen consumption by the difference in oxygen content between arterial and systemic venous blood, while pulmonary flow is estimated by relating oxygen consumption to the difference in oxygen content between pulmonary venous or wedge samples and pulmonary arterial blood. If both the systemic and pulmonary flows are calculated, the difference between them represents the volume of blood flowing through the intracardiac shunt. Alternatively, the difference in oxygen saturations is used to assess the ratio of pulmonary to systemic blood flow, the Q_p/Q_s ratio. Blood flow is inversely related to the ateriovenous oxygen content difference between the sites of sampling, and the relationship Q_p/Q_s is therefore expressed as:

$$\frac{(\text{Arterial} - \text{mixed venous}) \text{ oxygen saturation}}{(\text{Pulmonary venous} - \text{pulmonary arterial}) \text{ saturation}}$$

When there is no intracardiac shunt, the cardiac output can be determined by the dye or thermal dilution techniques. Catheter-tip electromagnetic flow probes are used occasionally but only provide a quantitative estimate of blood flow if the diameter of the vessel in which they are used can be measured accurately.

The resistance of a vascular bed can be calculated if the pressure drop across it and the blood flow through it are both known. The pulmonary vascular resistance in arbitrary units is defined as the difference between mean pulmonary arterial and mean left atrial pressures, divided by the pulmonary blood flow. If the mean left atrial pressure is unknown, a figure for 'total pulmonary resistance' can be calculated instead. This is the mean pulmonary arterial pressure divided by the pulmonary blood flow. The normal pulmonary vascular resistance is less than 2 units (less than 160 dynes sec cm^{-5}), and the normal total pulmonary resistance is less than 4 units (320 dynes sec cm^{-5}).

Value of angiocardiography

The chief indications for angiocardiography are to confirm abnormalities suggested during catheterisation and to demonstrate anatomical features which are not necessarily apparent as haemodynamic disturbances. The site of injection of the contrast material depends on the presumptive nature and location of the lesion and should be as close as possible to the structure under study so that a concentrated bolus can be followed before it is diluted. A test dose should be given first to confirm that the tip of the catheter is located correctly (p. 49).

Even minor degrees of valvular incompetence can be detected radiologically as can the presence, magnitude and direction of blood flow through intracardiac shunts. In addition, the shape of the cardiac chambers can be delineated, areas of dyskinesia can be identified, and the vigour with which the ventricles contract can be assessed. A quantitative assessment of stroke output and residual volume can be made by measuring the dimensions of the left ventricle on the appropriate frames of the angiogram, and assuming that a cross-section of the left ventricular cavity is oval in shape.

Pulmonary angiography is performed by injecting contrast medium directly into the main pulmonary artery. Selective catheterisation and angiography are the methods of choice for defining the anatomy of the coronary arteries, and for identifying sites of obstruction and the degree to which filling occurs from collateral tributaries distal to the obstruction.

SEDATION, ANALGESIA AND ANAESTHESIA FOR CARDIAC CATHETERISATION

The time taken to complete cardiac catheterisation and angiocardiography varies from 15 minutes to more than 2 hours. While it is in progress, the patient is required to lie still on a hard table in a room which at times is partially or completely darkened. Passage of the catheter is rarely painful but the proximity of the camera and recording apparatus may be disturbing. Angiocardiography is unpleasant because injection of the contrast material is followed by a sensation of warmth often accompanied by palpitations, nausea or even faintness. At the same time, attendants leave the patient's bedside to avoid unnecessary irradiation, and the noise level, which is usually considerable throughout, reaches a maximum.

Adult patients can generally tolerate these discomforts with only minimal sedation; 200 mg sodium amytal given by mouth 1 hour before catheterisation is often sufficient provided each event is explained carefully and the patient is reassured throughout. Local anaesthesia is required for the arterial and venous cut-downs and should be reinforced if necessary when the vessels are repaired. Increments of intravenous diazepam can be injected through the catheter if additional sedation is required while the procedure is in progress.

Heavier sedation or even general anaesthesia are required for cardiac catheterisation in uncooperative subjects, and particularly in infants and young children. Numerous techniques have been described, and their variety gives some indication of the fact that none is entirely satisfactory.

Two factors influence the choice of anaesthetic technique: the nature of the environment and the need to keep circulatory and respiratory function as stable and as near normal as possible. It has been noted already that some part of the procedure may be undertaken in a darkened room. This interferes with observation of the patient, but some security is provided by the ECG which is monitored continuously with both a visual display and an auditory warning. Intravascular pressures are displayed while the catheters are in place, and movement of both the heart and lungs can be seen while the patient is being screened. Other disadvantages of the catheterisation laboratory are that there is a profusion of electrical apparatus which precludes the use of explosive anaesthetic agents, access to the patient's head may be difficult, it may be necessary to tilt the table or move the patient along it, and finally, the anaesthetist may be exposed to unwanted irradiation.

The need for stable cardiorespiratory function is because measurements are made sequentially rather than simultaneously. The need for minimum interference with the performance of the heart, the pulmonary and peripheral vasculature, and with ventilation, is because these variables can all influence pressure, blood flow or oxygen saturation within the circulation. For example, the volume or even the direction of blood flow through an intracardiac shunt can be altered by changes in pulmonary or systemic vascular resistance: any fall in systemic vascular resistance encourages blood flow from right to left and the same is true if the pulmonary vascular resistance is elevated, or if the intrathoracic pressure is raised by artificial ventilation. Hypoxia and hypercapnia both increase the pulmonary vascular resistance, and not only influence blood flow through intracardiac shunts, but also increase the concentration of circulating catecholamines and predispose to cardiac dysrhythmias. Raising the inspired oxygen concentration may eliminate hypoxaemia but is undesirable because the volume of oxygen in solution will increase, so making it difficult to interpret small differences in oxygen saturation. High inspired oxygen concentrations can even be dangerous in neonates who are dependent on continued blood flow through a patent ductus arteriosus because the ductus will tend to close if the oxygen tension rises.

It should also be remembered that patients requiring cardiac catheterisation are suffering from significant cardiac disease which, in the vast majority of cases, can only be influenced adversely, if at all, by the investigation (an exception is Rashkind's balloon atrial septostomy, p. 176). This is in contrast with cardiac *surgery* in which correction or palliation of the haemodynamic disturbances is anticipated. An anaesthetic technique must be chosen which provides satisfactory conditions for the procedure but which does not add to the hazards.

Sedative techniques

Interference with cardiac or respiratory function is so likely to occur during general anaesthesia that heavy sedation, with the patient breathing spontaneously and inhaling room air, is often regarded as preferable. Unfortunately, this does not exclude the possibility of respiratory depression and many sedative drugs also affect the cardiovascular system. Apparently well-sedated children sometimes move unexpectedly in response to painful stimuli and there is less opportunity for immediately effective resuscitation if a crisis does occur.

Rectal thiopentone (50 mg/kg) was a common choice at one time but the results were unpredictable. The drug may not be retained or absorbed efficiently, and some children are so deeply sedated that respiratory depression, hypotension or respiratory obstruction occur. There is no analgesia if thiopentone is given alone, and restlessness and vomiting are fairly common during recovery.

The combination of pethidine, chlorpromazine and promethazine is widely used, particularly for infants (p. 157), but it may influence blood flow through intracardiac shunts because the changes which occur in the pulmonary and systemic vascular resistances are in opposite directions (systemic vascular resistance falls, pulmonary vascular resistance rises). The injection can be preceded by an oral barbiturate or, if given alone, can be followed at the time of catheterisation by intravenous diazepam (up to 1 mg/kg). The combination of Pethidine Co. followed by intravenous diazepam produces long-lasting tranquillity but there is an unacceptable degree of respiratory depression in some patients.

The combination of oral trimeprazine (2–4 mg/kg) 4 hours before catherisation, followed 3 hours later by intramuscular morphine sulphate (0·2 mg/kg) or papaveretum (0·3 mg/kg) with hyoscine (0·006 mg/kg) is another regime which is satisfactory in a high proportion of patients.

In recent years, ketamine has achieved widespread popularity. After atropine premedication, an initial dose of 10 mg/kg is given intramuscularly and subsequent doses of 1 mg/kg are given intravenously when necessary. The initial injection is followed by an increase in cardiac output, heart rate and systemic arterial blood pressure. The pulmonary arterial pressure rises too, but this probably reflects the increase in cardiac output rather than any direct effect on the pulmonary vascular resistance. These changes are caused by the liberation of endogenous catecholamines and can be minimised by premedication with droperidol. The haemodynamic effects are transitory and are barely detectable after 15 minutes; insignificant changes follow subsequent injections. Although it is sometimes claimed that protective reflexes are retained, this is not always the case and an anaesthetist should be present throughout. Transitory respiratory depression occurs initially and isolated cases of apnoea have been reported.

Neuroleptanalgesic drugs are sometimes chosen, the chief disadvantage being the reduction in both pulmonary and systemic vascular resistance which follows droperidol or phenoperidine. The doses advocated are droperidol 0·1 mg/kg, and phenoperidine 0·02–0·04 mg/kg, or 'Innovar' (droperidol 2·5 mg + fentanyl 0·05 mg in 1 ml) in a dose of 0·025–0·04 ml/kg. Some respiratory depression is inevitable, the peak effects on both the circulation and respiration occurring after 10 minutes. 'Althesin' by infusion has been advocated recently, but circulatory disturbances are common.

General anaesthetic techniques

General anaesthesia permits greater flexibility in management and can be used as a supplement to heavy sedation, or may be undertaken from the outset. When used to supplement a sedative technique, anaesthesia is usually induced immediately before angiography which is one of the most disturbing parts of the procedure. A short-acting barbiturate, or the inhalation of nitrous oxide, oxygen and halothane are satisfactory and intubation is unnecessary. Apnoea is required while the angiographic films are being exposed and an injection of suxamethonium preceded by atropine is all that is required; occasionally a request is made to hold the lungs inflated to slow the passage of contrast medium through the pulmonary circulation.

It is more difficult to provide a satisfactory general anaesthetic to supplement a sedative technique which has proved unsuccessful. Considerable respiratory depression may exist already, and the mouth, pharynx and stomach may be filled with sticky secretions if a young child has been sedated with chloral hydrate and then given a honey-coated dummy to suck. Intubation, taking all precautions to prevent contamination of the lungs with stomach contents, followed by controlled ventilation with 30–33% oxygen in nitrous oxide, is the best solution to this problem.

Cyanosis is common in cardiac disease, particularly in patients with congenital cardiac anomalies, and the temptation to use a high inspired oxygen concentration routinely 'because the patient is blue' should be avoided. It is usually possible to ensure full saturation of all blood passing through the lungs if the inspired oxygen concentration is 30–33%. Higher concentrations should only be used if there is definite pulmonary pathology too, or if the child's condition is critical. Occasionally, a request is made to use 100% oxygen for a short time; this is to determine whether an elevated pulmonary vascular resistance is fixed or labile—an increase in the inspired oxygen concentration will lower the pulmonary vascular resistance unless it is fixed. There is no longer any need to avoid nitrous oxide entirely because modern methods of oximetry are uninfluenced by the presence of this gas.

If general anaesthesia is to be used from the outset, there is a choice between spontaneous and controlled ventilation. Lightly premedicated subjects (e.g. trimeprazine, up to 4 mg/kg followed by atropine) usually ventilate adequately if allowed to breathe nitrous oxide and oxygen with low concentrations of halothane, but the cardiovascular effects of halothane are unacceptable in the frail or very young.

Controlled ventilation undoubtedly influences both the cardiac output and the ratio of pulmonary to systemic blood flow in the presence of intracardiac shunts. These effects are minimised if the arterial carbon dioxide tension is not lowered unduly and a consistent pattern of ventilation is used, aiming to keep the intrathoracic pressure as low as possible. Anaesthesia is induced with an intravenous barbiturate or with nitrous oxide, oxygen and halothane. Intubation is carried out with the aid of a muscle relaxant, and anaesthesia is continued with 30–33% oxygen in nitrous oxide and controlled ventilation. This is by far the easiest way of providing stable conditions with least hazard attributable to the anaesthetic agents. The conclusions drawn from the study provide a reliable indication of the nature and severity of the lesion and can be used safely to determine subsequent management. For these reasons, light general anaesthesia with controlled ventilation is widely regarded as the technique of choice.

COMPLICATIONS OF CARDIAC CATHETERISATION AND ANGIOCARDIOGRAPHY

The incidence of complications which can be attributed to cardiac catheterisation and angiography is closely related to the experience of the operator, and a mortality rate which is consistently less than 1% can be achieved by skilled staff. There are a number of hazards which, for convenience, are considered here under six headings.

Disturbances of blood volume

Blood loss during catheterisation can be considerable, particularly during arterial cannulation or while the vessel is being repaired. Hypovolaemia can also follow withdrawal of multiple blood samples, and conversely, fluid overload can occur if the catheters are flushed too frequently with large volumes of electrolyte solution. These hazards are, of course, much more important in infants.

Mechanical trauma

The vessels used for the introduction of cardiac catheters are damaged occasionally. Peripheral veins are often tied off when the catheter has been withdrawn and this can be inconvenient if the patient requires another study. Thrombophlebitis is sometimes seen but it generally resolves without active treatment and serious venous complications are rare.

Arterial damage is much more dangerous and occurs if tortuous vessels are perforated, if emboli form on the catheter and are disloged when it is withdrawn, if the artery is narrowed when the wall is repaired, or if the intima of the vessel is dissected during manipulation of a catheter which has not been introduced right into the arterial lumen. Ischaemia of distal tissues will result unless the patency of the vessel can be restored. The limb is cool and usually pale. The pulses are absent or barely palpable, and pain or weakness may be noticed, particularly during exercise; defective growth of the arm or leg can follow catheterisation of the axillary or femoral artery in infancy. In extreme cases, tissue necrosis occurs and damaged arteries should always be explored surgically to prevent this happening.

When the femoral artery has been catheterised percutaneously, pressure is applied after the catheter has been withdrawn and the bleeding usually stops quite quickly. This may not be so in hypertensive patients or those treated with anticoagulants. A haematoma forms, but although this is unsightly it is surprisingly painless unless the pressure is so great that the artery or adjacent vein are compressed.

Vascular damage is not restricted to peripheral vessels. The intrathoracic vessels or the myocardium can be punctured while the catheter is being manipulated. Cardiac tamponade can prove rapidly fatal if sudden haemorrhage occurs into the pericardial cavity, but there may be little bleeding if the atrial wall has been perforated. Further damage will result if contrast medium is injected into the myocardium or extravascularly and a test dose should always be given first. This should be cleared rapidly; persistent opacification suggests the tip of the catheter is lodged in the myocardium or is outside the heart. Anginal pain, dysrhythmias or hypotension follow intramyocardial injection and cardiac rupture has been reported.

An uncommon cause of vascular damage is catheterisation and angiography to demonstrate an aortic dissection. The thin wall of the aneurysm (arterial adventitia) can be torn very easily if the catheter enters the false lumen. This is particularly likely to occur during angiography when the aneurysm will either rupture, or the dissection will extend much further.

Dysrhythmias and myocardial infarction

Manipulation of catheters within the heart is a potent cause of dysrhythmias, particularly movement in the outflow tract of the left ventricle or catheterisation of the coronary arteries. Isolated extrasystoles are often ignored, but the catheter should be moved, or withdrawn into a proximal chamber if dysrhythmias persist, especially if runs of ventricular extrasystoles are seen. The usual drugs must be available to treat rhythm disturbances, particularly atropine and lignocaine. Ventricular fibrillation or asystole sometimes occur unexpectedly and resuscitation equipment must always be available. Resuscitation is usually successful, but if a satisfactory circulation cannot be restored easily the possibility of cardiac tamponade, myocardial infarction or serious haemorrhage should be considered.

Myocardial infarction is a recognised complication of coronary arterial catheterisation and angiography. The wall of the vessel can be dissected by the tip of the catheter or by the force of injection during angiography, plaques of atheroma can be dislodged and impacted in the lumen, and the slow passage of a bolus of contrast medium through narrowed vessels can provoke serious coronary ischaemia with subsequent hypotension and infarction.

Adverse reactions to contrast media

Modern contrast media are relatively non-toxic but adverse reactions do still occur and may be related to hypersensitivity of the patient or to the sodium content or hypertonicity of the solutions. The risks of myocardial infarction complicating coronary angiography, and the mechanical hazards of intramyocardial injection have been noted already.

All contrast media cause a reduction in systemic vascular resistance, an increase in pulmonary vascular resistance and are directly depressant to the myocardium. The reduction in systemic vascular resistance accounts for the sensations of warmth, nausea and faintness; hypotension is usually observed and dysrhythmias can be provoked by the combination of hypotension and myocardial depression. Hypertension is seen occasionally and may represent a reaction to pain or fear, or a sudden increase in intravascular volume caused by the hypertonic injectate.

The increase in pulmonary vascular resistance which follows injection into the right heart or pulmonary artery is relatively unimportant if the pulmonary vascular bed is normal. Acute right heart failure or asystole can occur if the pulmonary vascular resistance is already elevated; complications are particularly likely to occur during pulmonary angiography in patients suffering from pulmonary embolic disease because the increase in pulmonary vascular resistance is accompanied by a fall in systemic resistance, while the cardiac output is already low and cannot increase.

Acute pulmonary oedema may develop, for example in patients with mitral stenosis, because the injection of hypertonic contrast medium causes an abrupt increase in the pulmonary blood volume if flow through the pulmonary circulation is slow.

Convulsions and clouding of consciousness have been reported following angiocardiography, but are now rare. The aetiology is not entirely clear but may be cerebral oedema caused by capillary damage which occurs when repeated injections of contrast medium reach the cerebral circulation in high concentration. Cerebral venous thrombosis is an occasional complication in polycythaemic, cyanosed infants and should be suspected if recovery from general anaesthesia is unduly prolonged. Treatment is with intravenous fluid infusion and possibly thrombolytic drugs.

Embolism

Blood clot, air bubbles, or segments of fractured catheters or guide wires can all cause systemic embolism; occasionally, fragments of atheroma, calcium, or intracardiac clot are dislodged into the circulation. The incidence of thrombosis or embolism related to arterial catheterisation is decreased by anticoagulation with heparin. Air embolism is avoided by ensuring that the transducer and catheter system is filled with saline, that the syringes used for flushing are kept vertical, that bubbles are not introduced when blood samples are withdrawn, and above all, that air is eliminated from the syringes and pump used for angiography.

Miscellaneous complications

A number of complications cannot be classified under the preceding headings. Such adverse features include hypothermia in infancy, haemorrhage related to coagulation defects which are also more common in premature infants, and bacterial endocarditis developing in the postcatheterisation period if infection is introduced at the time of the study. Catheters are sometimes tied into knots within the cardiac cavities. They can generally be untied by rotating the catheter to free the loop, or the knot can be withdrawn into the peripheral vessel where it is removed by enlarging the vascular incision. Finally, it must not be forgotten that there is a mortality and morbidity related to general anaesthesia for cardiac catheterisation.

NON-INVASIVE CARDIODIAGNOSTIC TECHNIQUES

Echocardiography

The application of a high frequency alternating current to a piezoelectric crystal causes it to vibrate and produce ultrasonic pulses. These traverse tissues but are reflected at the interface between structures of different acoustic impedance. This reflected energy or 'echo' is returned to the piezoelectric crystal and so transduced into an electrical signal which can be amplified and recorded. The transducer is applied to the chest wall in such a way that the beam of ultrasonic pulses is approximately perpendicular to the structure under study and does not pass through the lungs. Echoes can be reflected from the surfaces of the heart, the septum and the leaflets of the mitral valve and are generally recorded photographically. The technique is of particular value for diagnosing mitral valve disease or the presence of a pericardial effusion, and intracardiac tumours can be delineated. The functional state of the ventricles can be assessed by noting the movement of the ventricular walls and septum, and quantitative methods have been developed for calculating the ventricular volume and stroke output. The method is being evaluated as a means of diagnosing congenital heart disease but is unlikely to replace cardiac catheterisation in this field.

Other non-invasive methods of investigation such as phonocardiography, apex cardiography, analysis of the carotid arterial waveform, and impedance cardiography are sometimes used to supplement cardiac catheterisation, but they rarely provide information which is of relevance to cardiac surgery. A technique which may prove invaluable in the future is cardiological diagnosis by means of an ECG-linked whole body scanner.

REFERENCES

PRINCIPLES OF CARDIAC CATHETERISATION AND ANGIOCARDIOGRAPHY

MILLER H. C., BROWN D. J. & MILLER G. A. H. (1974) A comparison of formulae used to estimate oxygen saturation in mixed venous blood from caval samples. *British Heart Journal* **36,** 446.

VEREL D. (1971) Diagnostic procedures available for the investigation of patients with cardiac disease. *British Journal of Anaesthesia* **43,** 268.

VEREL D. & GRAINGER R. G. (1969) *Cardiac Catheterization and Angiocardiography: an introductory manual.* E & S Livingstone, Edinburgh.

YANG S. Y., BENTIVOGLIO L. G., MARANHAO V. & GOLDBERG H. (1972) From *Cardiac Catheterization Data to Hemodynamic Parameters.* F. A. Davis Company, Philadelphia.

ANAESTHESIA FOR CARDIAC CATHETERISATION

ALDERSON J. D., HAMPSON J. M., JEBSON P. J. R. & THORNTON J. A. (1976) Althesin infusion for cardiac catheterisation. *Anaesthesia* **31,** 280.

COPPEL D. L. & DUNDEE J. W. (1972) Ketamine anaesthesia for cardiac catheterisation. *Anaesthesia* **27,** 25.

GASSNER S., COHEN M., AYGEN M., LEVY E., VENTURA E. & SHASHDI J. (1974) The effect of ketamine on pulmonary artery pressure: an experimental and clinical study. *Anaesthesia* **29,** 141.

GOLDBERG S. J., LINDE L. M., WOLFE R. R., GRISWOLD W. & MOMMA K. (1969) The effects of meperidine, promethazine and chlorpromazine on pulmonary and systemic circulation. *American Heart Journal* **77,** 214.

HEALY T. E. J. (1969) Intravenous diazepam for cardiac catheterisation. *Anaesthesia* **24,** 537.

MACDONALD H. R., BRAID D. P., STEAD B. R., CRAWFORD I. C. & TAYLOR S. H. (1966) Clinical and circulatory effects of neuroleptanalgesia with dehydrobenzperidol and phenoperidine. *British Heart Journal* **28,** 654.

MANNERS J. M. & CODMAN V. A. (1969) General anaesthesia for cardiac catheterisation in children. The effect of spontaneous or controlled ventilation on the evaluation of congenital abnormalities. *Anaesthesia* **24,** 541.

MANNERS J. M. (1971) Anaesthesia for diagnostic procedures in cardiac disease. *British Journal of Anaesthesia* **43,** 276.

MOFFITT E. A., McGOON D. W. & RITTER D. G. (1970) The diagnosis and correction of congenital cardiac defects. *Anesthesiology* **33,** 144.

NICHOLSON J. R. & GRAHAM G. R. (1969) Management of infants under six months of age undergoing cardiac investigation. *British Journal of Anaesthesia* **41,** 417.

TARHAN S., MOFFITT E. A., LUNDBORG R. O. & FRYE R. L. (1971) Hemodynamic and blood-gas effects of Innovar in patients with acquired heart disease. *Anesthesiology* **34,** 250.

TWEED W. A., MINUCK M. & MYMIN D. (1972) Circulatory responses to ketamine anesthesia. *Anesthesiology* **37,** 613.

NON-INVASIVE CARDIODIAGNOSTIC TECHNIQUES

GIBSON D. G. (1975) The assessment of left ventricular function in man by non-invasive techniques. In *Modern Trends in Cardiology* **3,** Ed. M. F. Oliver, p. 247. Butterworth, London.

Leading Article (1974) Ultrasounding the heart. *British Medical Journal* **1,** 83.

NAGGAR C. Z., DOBNIK D. B., FLESSAS A. P., KRIPKE B. J. & RYAN T. J. (1975) Accuracy of the stroke index as determined by the transthoracic electrical impedance method. *Anesthesiology* **42,** 201.

RASSMUSSEN J. P., SØRENSEN B. & KANN T. (1975) Evaluation of impedance cardiography as a non-invasive means of measuring systolic time intervals and cardiac output. *Acta Anaesthesiologica Scandinavica* **19,** 210.

CHAPTER 5

ANAESTHESIA FOR CLOSED CARDIAC PROCEDURES

General considerations governing anaesthetic management
Closed mitral valvotomy
Anaesthetic management
Closure of patent ductus arteriosus
Anaesthetic management
Resection of coarctation of the aorta
Anaesthetic management
Left atrio-femoral bypass

Pericardial disease
Anaesthetic management—cardiac tamponade
Anaesthetic management—constrictive pericarditis
Insertion of pacemakers
Anaesthetic management
Cardioversion

The term 'closed' cardiac surgery refers to operations which are performed without the support of cardiopulmonary bypass. It is customary to include surgery of the great vessels as well as operations on the heart itself, and several 'closed' procedures, particularly those carried out in infancy or childhood, are purely palliative.

GENERAL CONSIDERATIONS GOVERNING ANAESTHETIC MANAGEMENT

Cardiac surgery always entails thoracotomy. Although acupuncture analgesia and spontaneous ventilation have been used successfully, conventional anaesthetic management requires endotracheal intubation and controlled ventilation. Light general anaesthesia is sufficient because surgical stimulation is relatively slight once the chest has been opened.

Thiopentone can be used safely for induction in almost every case. The drug is rapid in effect, totally predictable, and there is an extremely low incidence of hypersensitivity reactions, abnormalities of muscle tone or disturbances of ventilation. It is sometimes stated that thiopentone should not be given to patients with cardiac disease because the combination of myocardial depression and a reduction in systemic vascular resistance can cause hypotension. However, part of the mechanism of hypotension following thiopentone is a reduction in venous tone, and hence in ventricular filling and stroke output. Two features of the circulation in heart failure lessen the risk of hypotension from this cause. In the first place, the blood volume is elevated in chronic

54

heart failure and the systemic veins are often engorged. Changes in venous tone therefore have less effect on cardiac filling than in normal subjects. Secondly, the performance of the failing heart is influenced far less by changes in filling pressure than the normal myocardium (p. 5).

The reduction in systemic arterial tone cannot be dismissed so lightly. There is little change in the output from a normal heart when the arterial resistance is lowered slightly, but a reflex increase in stroke volume occurs if the arterial resistance falls considerably. When the heart is failing, stroke work is limited. A modest reduction in systemic vascular resistance (after-load) permits an increase in stroke volume at the expense of the pressure generated. Within limits, this may be advantageous; however, the stroke volume cannot increase if the ventricle cannot fill readily (e.g. tight mitral stenosis) or if myocardial function is depressed by a lowered perfusion pressure.

In practice, a sleep dose of thiopentone is well tolerated by patients pre-senting for elective surgery, provided the injection is given slowly to allow for the prolonged circulation time which is so often a feature of cardiac disease. Alternative induction agents are intravenous diazepam or a neurolep-tic combination such as droperidol and fentanyl (p. 77).

Preoxygenation is desirable for patients with pulmonary sequelae, for those with a limited cardiac output, or those who are prone to dysrhythmias. An inhalational induction is rarely ideal except for patients with the tetralogy of Fallot (p. 123). It tends to cause anxiety and is often slow, there is a risk of hypoxia if anaesthetic concentrations of nitrous oxide are used, and irrita-tion of the respiratory tract, dysrhythmias or hypotension are likely to accom-pany ether, cyclopropane or halothane.

Spontaneous ventilation can generally be resumed immediately after closed cardiac surgery, and muscle relaxants which can be reversed at the end of operation are preferable to large doses of central respiratory depressant drugs (cf. open heart surgery, p. 77).

Either short- or long-acting relaxants can be used to provide good condi-tions for endotracheal intubation, although theoretically the effective dose of suxamethonium reaching the end-plates is decreased when the circulation time is prolonged. The duration of most cardiac surgical procedures is such that if long-acting relaxants are chosen, a fully paralysing dose can be given at the time of induction without creating a risk of residual paralysis in the postoperative period. The choice of non-depolarising agents eliminates the possible hazard of dysrhythmias provoked by suxamethonium and avoids any disturbance to the lightly anaesthetised patient during the transition between short- and long-acting drugs. At the present time, pancuronium bro-mide is probably the non-depolarising agent of choice, even though it tends to cause an increase in heart rate. D-tubocurarine and gallamine triethiodide are both undesirable, the former because occasional patients develop profound hypotension and the latter because of the inevitable tachycardia. If intubation is carried out using a long-acting drug, it is essential to assist and then to control ventilation while awaiting the onset of complete relaxation. Use of a mixture of nitrous oxide and oxygen prevents the return of consciousness following the relatively small dose of thiopentone. There is no need to spray the trachea with local anaesthetic and intubation can generally be carried out so quickly that inflation with oxygen prior to this manœuvre is unnecessary.

Thoracotomy in the lateral position is a common requirement, and ventilation to the upper lung may be restricted. This is rarely a problem during surgery on the descending aorta but considerable retraction of the upper lung is necessary if access to the heart, ascending aorta or pulmonary artery is required. Some ventilation to this side is possible and an endobronchial anaesthetic technique is only indicated very occasionally, e.g. during the resection of an extensive aneurysm of the thoracic aorta, involving the lung or pleural cavity. The pattern of controlled ventilation is generally not of critical importance during closed cardiac surgery, and the mechanical effects of intermittent positive pressure ventilation on the circulation are minimal once the chest has been opened.

Anaesthesia can be maintained with nitrous oxide and oxygen and this combination is advocated by most practising anaesthetists although even nitrous oxide has been incriminated as a myocardial depressant. 35–40% oxygen is recommended to minimise the risk of hypoxaemia caused either by pulmonary abnormalities or by retraction of the lung during exposure of the heart.

Narcotic or analgesic supplements are only needed in small doses. Opiates are preferable to pethidine because there is less change in blood pressure or pulse rate; phenoperidine or fentanyl are effective but sometimes cause unexpected hypotension or muscular rigidity.

Haemorrhage is always a hazard, and an intravenous infusion using a wide-bore cannula is essential; facilities for warming the transfused blood should always be available. It is sometimes desirable to site the cannula so that the central venous pressure can be monitored, but a number of the more straightforward procedures, e.g. resection of aortic coarctation or closure of a patent ductus arteriosus, can be undertaken safely without this. Blood loss can be assessed by measuring the volume accumulating in the suction apparatus and by swab weighing.

The ECG and arterial blood pressure are monitored routinely but intra-arterial cannulation and continuous display of the pressure are only required occasionally; these instances are mentioned individually. Catheterisation of the bladder and monitoring of body temperature are not required during closed cardiac surgery in adults. The only other essential prerequisite is that resuscitation equipment, including a DC defibrillator, must be ready in the operating theatre, not merely available within the theatre suite.

CLOSED MITRAL VALVOTOMY

The chest is opened through a left anterolateral incision and the fused commissures of the mitral valve are split with a dilator which is introduced through the left ventricle and guided by the surgeon's finger in the left atrium. The advent of open heart surgery has decreased the popularity of closed valvotomy because the anatomy of the valve can only be assessed by palpation, the degree and direction of splitting may be difficult to control, and there is a risk of systemic embolism if clot is present in the left atrium or if the valve is calcified. The procedure is reserved for patients with pure mitral stenosis and mobile valve cusps, features which are indicated clinically by a full-length diastolic murmur and a loud opening snap. These criteria are generally only fulfilled by relatively young patients who have not developed much, if any, pulmonary vascular disease.

The presence of the stenosed valve means that the left ventricle can only fill slowly; the cardiac output is low and fails to rise normally in response to an increased demand. The arm to brain circulation time is prolonged because of the low output and increased central blood volume.

Optimal left ventricular filling requires a slow heart rate with a long diastolic interval as well as a considerable head of pressure in the left atrium; left atrial systole contributes significantly when sinus rhythm is present. Left ventricular filling will be impaired and the cardiac output will fall if hypovolaemia lowers the left atrial pressure, if diastole is shortened by the development of a tachycardia, or if the benefit of atrial systole is lost because of the onset of a dysrhythmia. Rhythm or rate changes are particularly hazardous because there is both a reduction in ventricular filling and an increase in left atrial pressure; pulmonary oedema may occur as a result. Peripheral vasodilatation is also dangerous because the limited filling of the left ventricle prevents any increase in stroke volume in response to the reduction in afterload. Attempts to restore the blood pressure by transfusion are unlikely to succeed but will merely increase the already elevated left atrial pressure.

Anaesthetic management

Generous sedative premedication is particularly important to avoid the tachycardia of anxiety. Patients who are orthopnoeic should be brought to the operating theatre supported on several pillows. The arrival of a restless, agitated patient with a tachycardia and dry cough indicates that premedication has been inadequate and that acute pulmonary oedema is imminent. If this should occur, it is advisable to proceed immediately with oxygenation, induction and artificial ventilation. This is generally sufficient to cause redistribution of blood away from the engorged pulmonary circulation without causing a prohibitive reduction in cardiac output. In spite of the theoretical considerations outlined above, a sleep dose of thiopentone can be given safely.

The operation entails considerable manipulation of the heart. Rhythm disturbances and hypotension are common, and it is desirable to record both the blood pressure and central venous pressure continuously using an intra-arterial cannula and centrally situated intravenous infusion.

Unless there are dense adhesions, for example following previous valvo-

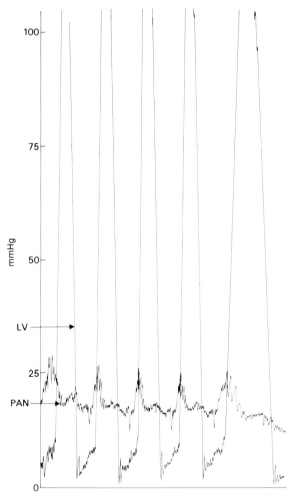

Figure 5.1 Mitral stenosis: male age 40. Left ventricular and pulmonary arterial 'wedge' pressures with a mean gradient of 11 mm Hg (1·5 kPa) across the mitral valve. The right heart pressures were only slightly elevated (right ventricle 36/2 mm Hg; 4·8/0·3 kPa), and the pulmonary vascular resistance was normal. A minor degree of mitral regurgitation was demonstrated on angiography.

tomy, blood transfusion may not be required initially but the infusion should be changed to whole blood before the heart is opened. The mitral valve is assessed by palpation and by simultaneously recording pressures in the left atrium and left ventricle. An end-diastolic pressure gradient is characteristic of mitral stenosis (Fig. 5.1) but it may be trivial in spite of severe stenosis if the cardiac output is very low when the measurements are made. There is virtually no cardiac output while the valve is being palpated and it is desirable to allow a short recovery period after assessment. Blood loss is replaced if necessary and several hundred ml may be required if blood has been intentionally allowed to escape through the atrial incision to sweep out blood clot. When systemic embolism is a particular hazard, some surgeons elect to place snares around the innominate and carotid arteries and occlude these while the valve is being opened. The period of occlusion should be timed carefully, but is generally short. As an alternative, the anaesthetist may be requested to apply pressure to both carotid arteries in the neck, but it is extremely difficult to do this effectively when the patient is in the semi-lateral position. The mitral valve is occluded again during the valvotomy and the left ventricle is disturbed too. Ventricular extrasystoles are common and it is wise to provide a few breaths of 100% oxygen immediately beforehand to ensure that any blood reaching the coronary arteries is fully oxygenated.

The pulse often returns rapidly after the valvotomy, but sometimes a short period of ventricular support is needed; bolus doses of isoprenaline (1–3 μg) are usually sufficient. Once the circulation appears stable, the state of the valve is reassessed to determine whether there is any residual mitral stenosis or regurgitation. Provided a satisfactory valvotomy has been achieved, the remainder of the procedure should be uneventful; transfusion is continued to replace blood loss, but prolonged monitoring of the left atrial pressure is not required. Adequate spontaneous ventilation can almost always be restored at the end of the operation and the patient is returned to the Intensive Care Unit breathing oxygen-enriched air.

CLOSURE OF PATENT DUCTUS ARTERIOSUS

When the ductus arteriosus remains patent, blood flows from the aorta into the lower resistance of the pulmonary circulation and causes pulmonary plethora. If the flow through the ductus is particularly large or if there are other congenital anomalies present, pulmonary oedema may occur in infancy. More commonly, the child is symptom-free and a murmur is heard during routine medical examination. If diagnosis is delayed until the patient is adult, there may be pulmonary or pulmonary vascular sequelae (p. 18) which in some cases contraindicate closure.

Anaesthetic management

The procedure is carried out through a left thoracotomy but there is little interference with ventilation to the left lung because the surgical approach is posterior. In uncomplicated cases, there are no particular restraints on the choice of premedication, induction technique or maintenance of anaesthesia, apart from the need to ensure that there is no coughing or straining while the aortic and pulmonary ends of the ductus are being secured. If the ductus is particularly tense, a request is sometimes made for systemic hypotension while the vessels are being dissected. The blood pressure can be monitored satisfactorily with a sphygmomanometer, using a cuff on the right arm because control of the ductus may involve temporary clamping of the left subclavian artery. The operation can often be completed without blood transfusion, but haemorrhage is a major hazard, particularly if the ductus is short and wide, or if it is calcified. A rare complication is damage to the recurrent laryngeal nerve.

In very occasional circumstances, it is necessary to use left atriofemoral bypass so that the aorta can be cross-clamped above and below the site of the ductus. This procedure is described in detail on p. 63.

Patients with a patent ductus arteriosus complicated by pulmonary hypertension and a bidirectional shunt (p. 18) are occasionally submitted to thoracotomy to assess the feasibility of closing the ductus. Hypoxia and hypercarbia must be avoided with particular care because both increase the pulmonary vascular resistance and accentuate the right to left shunt. After the ductus has been mobilised, it is occluded for a trial period while pressures are recorded in the aorta and pulmonary artery. If closure is feasible, clamping the ductus results in an increase in systemic and fall in pulmonary arterial pressure, but the reverse is true if the pulmonary vascular resistance is high and fixed. This indicates that the condition is inoperable; the ductus is released and the chest is closed leaving the haemodynamic abnormality uncorrected. Patients with pulmonary vascular disease are prone to postoperative respiratory and circulatory complications and may need a period of artificial ventilation.

RESECTION OF COARCTATION OF THE AORTA

The coarctation can be proximal or distal to the site of the ductus arteriosus. A preductal coarctation is often a long narrow segment rather than an isolated stricture and other important congenital cardiac anomalies commonly coexist. These cases generally present with left ventricular failure in infancy.

Postductal coarctation may remain undetected for a number of years. Numerous collateral vessels develop between arteries arising from the aorta proximal and distal to the stricture, largely through internal mammary and intercostal anastomoses. These alleviate both the proximal hypertension and the relative ischaemia of tissues distal to the stricture and are responsible for the characteristic 'rib notching' which is visible on the chest X-ray (Figure 5.2). In spite of the collaterals, the pressure in the upper limbs remains elevated and is often greater on the right than the left because the left subclavian artery is involved in the coarctation. In time, untreated proximal hypertension results in left ventricular hypertrophy and patients present with anginal pain or the dyspnoea of left ventricular failure. The incidence of subarachnoid haemorrhage is increased because there is an association between coarctation, and berry aneurysms on the circle of Willis which are likely to rupture because the blood pressure is elevated. Dissection of the aorta occurs occasionally

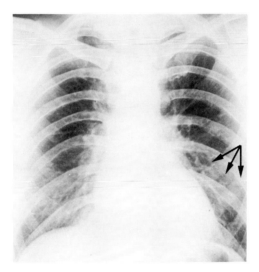

Figure 5.2 Extensive rib notching in a man of 34 years with coarctation of the aorta; this is seen most clearly at the site of the arrows.

and may involve the aortic valve. The aortic valve is sometimes bicuspid and may be the site of subacute bacterial endocarditis; this is more common than infection at the site of the coarctation.

Three problems warrant specific attention during anaesthesia for resection of coarctation. The first is haemorrhage which occurs while the chest is being opened and the coarctation mobilised. It originates from numerous collateral vessels which are perfused at high pressure, and it can be controlled to some extent if a hypotensive technique is employed.

The second problem is the increase in proximal hypertension which results when the aorta is cross-clamped above and below the stricture. If the coarctation is moderately severe and the collateral vessels are well developed, the rise in blood pressure is no more than 30–50 mm Hg (4·0–6·7 kPa). This can be tolerated unless the patient suffers from left ventricular failure or aortic incompetence, or has a past history of cerebrovascular accident. If the coarctation is relatively mild and few collaterals have developed, severe proximal hypertension will occur. It is important to note that this is not amenable to control by hypotensive agents once the aorta has been clamped. Vasodilatation in the territory supplied by the first two or three branches from the aorta will do little to reduce the pressure when virtually the entire cardiac output is being delivered into these vessels. Hypotensive drugs given while the aorta is cross-clamped will however dilate the vessels in the rest of the body, and undesirable hypotension is likely to occur when the aortic clamps are released.

The third and final problem is also a feature of relatively mild coarctation, namely ischaemia of tissues supplied by vessels arising from the aorta distal to the stricture. Although it might be anticipated that the kidneys are most vulnerable, it is the spinal cord which is most at risk. It may be necessary to divide a number of intercostal arteries while the coarctation is being mobilised, and this interupts the segmental supply to the cord. If there are inadequate collaterals or the anterior spinal artery is particularly small, ischaemia of the cord can occur and result in paraplegia.

Anaesthetic management

The operation is carried out through a left posterolateral thoracotomy; premedication and the induction of anaesthesia are straightforward unless cardiovascular or cerebral complications are present. It is essential to monitor the arterial pressure on the right arm because the left subclavian artery is virtually always clamped while the aortic resection is in progress. Intra-arterial pressure monitoring is rarely required, even if a hypotensive technique is to be employed because lowering the pressure to less than 80–100 mm Hg (10·6–13·3 kPa) is neither necessary nor is it generally feasible.

An infusion of sodium nitroprusside or of 0·1% trimetaphan camphorsulphate produces rapidly reversible hypotension. The rate at which the drug is given may vary if the same intravenous route is used for blood transfusion and separate infusion sites are sometimes recommended. Alternatively, an attempt can be made to induce hypotension by vigorous positive pressure ventilation with halothane, but this is often ineffective in healthy subjects. The hypotensive technique is initiated before the commencement of surgery and is discontinued just before the aortic clamps are applied.

Resection of the coarctation and repair of the aorta are generally complete in 30 to 60 minutes. The vessels in the lower half of the body are less well perfused than normal during this time, but a metabolic acidosis does not occur and infusion of sodium bicarbonate is not required. When the aortic repair is complete the clamps are cautiously removed; the blood pressure falls but not profoundly unless there is unexpected haemorrhage from the suture line.

Two postoperative complications are worthy of note. The first is systemic hypertension which is particularly undesirable in the presence of a recently completed aortic suture line. Satisfactory control of the blood pressure can often be achieved by nursing the patient sitting upright and providing generous sedation. Chlorpromazine (10–25 mg) is particularly effective because sedation is combined with α-adrenergic blockade. If these measures are ineffective, an infusion of trimetaphan camphorsulphonate or other short-acting hypotensive agent can be considered.

The other unexpected postoperative complication is abdominal pain, possibly caused by exposure of the gastrointestinal tract to normal systolic and pulse pressures for the first time. Although the pain is sometimes severe and may be accompanied by paralytic ileus, there are generally no localising signs and the condition resolves spontaneously.

LEFT ATRIOFEMORAL BYPASS

This is the technique of choice for operations on the descending thoracic aorta in patients in whom aortic cross-clamping would cause intolerable proximal hypertension. While the aorta is clamped, oxygenated blood is drained from the left atrium and returned to the femoral artery at a flow rate which is adjusted to keep the mean femoral and radial arterial pressures approximately equal. The indications for using the technique include the relief of severe coarctation in patients who cannot tolerate even a slight increase in proximal hypertension (e.g. those with a history of heart failure or cerebrovascular accident), resection of a relatively mild coarctation when collateral vessels are poorly developed, the repair of a dissection, aneurysm or rupture of a previously normal descending aorta, and during surgery on the ductus arteriosus, or an otherwise uncomplicated coarctation, if unusual anatomical difficulties are anticipated.

Moment to moment changes in the arterial blood pressure are common, and it is therefore preferable to monitor the proximal aortic pressure using an intra-arterial cannula which must be situated in the *right* radial artery.

The patient is positioned so that there is easy access to the left groin as well as to the thoracotomy site. Heparin (3 mg/kg) is given when dissection of both the femoral artery and aorta is complete, and cannulae are then inserted into the left atrium and left femoral artery. These are joined through an extracorporeal circuit which consists of a reservoir and arterial pump together with suitable filters and a heat exchanger. Drainage from the left atrium is by gravity, so that air is not entrained in the circuit, and the blood

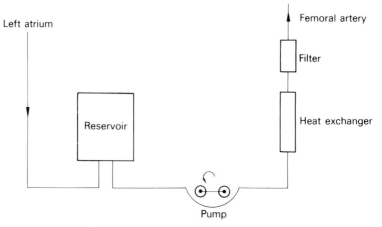

Left atrium

Femoral artery

Filter

Heat exchanger

Reservoir

Pump

Figure 5.3   Circuit diagram for left atriofemoral bypass.

is pumped back from the reservoir into the femoral artery. Bypass is discontinued at the end of the aortic repair, the left atrial cannula is removed, and the heparin is reversed with protamine sulphate (6 mg/kg).

PERICARDIAL DISEASE— RELIEF OF TAMPONADE AND CONSTRICTIVE PERICARDITIS

Cardiac tamponade exists when the pericardial sac is distended to such an extent that the heart is compressed and unable to fill. The distension is generally caused by fluid which may be serous, haemorrhagic or purulent. The haemodynamic consequences are the same whatever the nature of the fluid unless the tamponade develops as a complication of intrathoracic haemorrhage. This can occur following open heart surgery and is discussed in greater detail in Chapter 10.

Constrictive pericarditis is the term used when non-distensible, fibrous or calcified tissue surrounds and is adherent to the heart. The pericardium and its cavity cannot be identified, and fibrosis generally extends deeply into the myocardium. Sometimes, only part of the circumference of the heart is affected.

Cardiac tamponade and constrictive pericarditis impede ventricular filling; pulsus paradoxus, an accentuation of the normal inspiratory fall in systemic arterial blood pressure, is a feature of both (Fig. 5.4). There are at least two mechanisms contributing to this inspiratory reduction in stroke output and arterial blood pressure. In the first place, the effective filling gradient of the left ventricle (pulmonary wedge minus intrapericardial or intraventricular pressure), decreases on inspiration. This is because the intrathoracic and

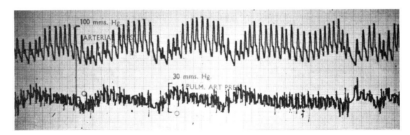

Figure 5.4 Pulsus paradoxus in a patient with constrictive pericarditis (spontaneous ventilation). The pressure measurements are referred to zero at the sternal angle.

hence the pulmonary venous pressures drop, whereas the intrapericardial or intraventricular pressure is little affected (Fig. 5.5). As a result, stroke volume and arterial blood pressure fall. Secondly, right ventricular filling is enhanced during inspiration, so restricting the space available for the left ventricle in the distended pericardial sac.

Cardiac tamponade and constrictive pericarditis both cause elevation of

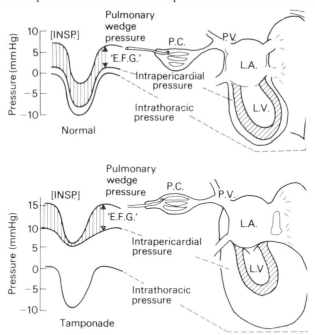

Figure 5.5 Changes in pulmonary wedge pressure, intrapericardial pressure and hence in effective filling gradient (EFG) of the left ventricle when the intrathoracic pressure varies with respiration. The normal situation is depicted in the upper half of the figure and the findings in cardiac tamponade in the lower half. Reproduced from Sharp *et al.*, 1960, by permission of the Editor, *American Journal of Medicine.*

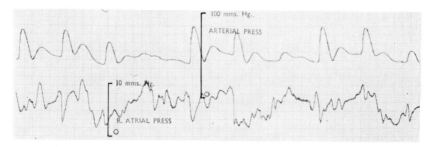

Figure 5.6 Cardiac tamponade: male aged 28. Systolic descent in the right atrial pressure; pulsus paradoxus is apparent in the arterial blood pressure. Pressure measurements are referred to zero at the sternal angle.

the atrial pressures, and the right atrial pressure will rise further during inspiration if blood drawn into the great veins cannot be accommodated in the heart. However, the waveform of the venous pressure differs between cardiac tamponade and chronic constrictive pericarditis. When the heart is surrounded by fluid, changes in pressure in the pericardial sac can be freely transmitted in all directions. The pressure in the pericardium will fall during ventricular systole when the heart decreases in size, and this is reflected by a systolic descent ('x' descent) in the right atrial pressure (Fig. 5.6). When the ventricle is surrounded by rigid tissue, the gradient from atria to ventricles is very high at the onset of ventricular diastole, and for a short while blood flows rapidly through the atrioventricular valves. This causes a rapid rise in pressure in the rigid ventricular cavities and blood flow soon slows. There is therefore a transitory postsystolic drop ('y' descent) in the atrial pressure (Fig. 5.7). The short-lived rapid flow of blood into the rigid ventricular cavity is probably also responsible for the loud third heart sound which is heard characteristically at the apex in patients suffering from chronic constrictive pericarditis.

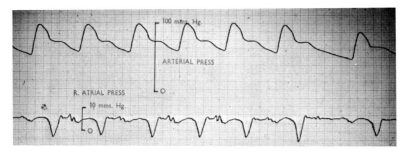

Figure 5.7 Constrictive pericarditis: male aged 36. Post-systolic descent in the right atrial pressure. Arterial paradox in this patient is shown in Fig. 5.4. Pressure measurements are referred to zero at the sternal angle.

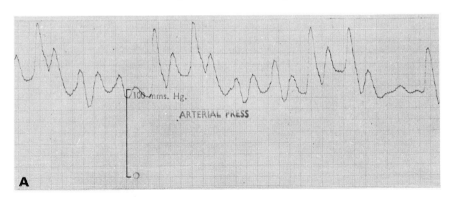

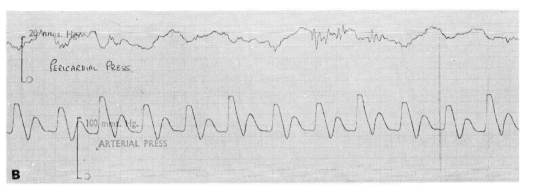

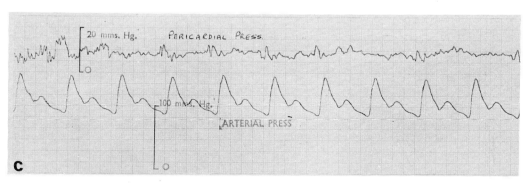

Figure 5.8 Cardiac tamponade, female aged 13 years.

A, The arterial blood pressure prior to the induction of anaesthesia;
B, The arterial and intrapericardial pressures following the induction of anaes-
thesia and during controlled ventilation with a 'tight' bag;
C, The same pressures after the aspiration of 280 ml of pericardial fluid.

All pressure measurements are referred to zero at the sternal angle.

Anaesthetic management—cardiac tamponade

Surgery is sometimes required to relieve cardiac tamponade and to establish a diagnosis. If the effusion is tense and the patient is acutely breathless or hypotensive, paracentesis should be undertaken first. If this is impossible, pre-medication with a small dose of atropine or hyoscine followed by induction with intravenous diazepam is preferable to thiopentone because even a slight reduction in ventricular filling pressure will cause a profound reduction in the cardiac output. Controlled ventilation is necessary, and should be instituted cautiously because it too may impede ventricular filling. Sometimes however, the intrapericardial pressure is so high that it is virtually un-influenced by intrathoracic pressure, and an increase in the absolute value of the pulmonary wedge pressure caused by positive pressure ventilation may actually augment ventricular filling and improve the output. Furthermore, if positive pressure ventilation impedes right ventricular filling, this will allow the left ventricle to fill more readily (see Fig. 5.8 and discussion on pulsus paradoxus, p. 64).

Anaesthetic management—constrictive pericarditis

Patients with constrictive pericarditis develop symptoms more insidiously than those with cardiac tamponade. They complain of fatigue, abdominal distension (ascites) and peripheral oedema rather than of dyspnoea. At operation, which is generally carried out through a median sternotomy, the thickened pericardial tissue is removed piecemeal. It is often impossible to clear the heart completely and a good functional result can generally be obtained without disturbing the more inaccessible surfaces. Postoperatively, the haemodynamic abnormalities resolve only slowly.

Haemorrhage during dissection of the adherent, thickened pericardial tissue is inevitable. It is not uncommon for the heart to be opened inadvertently, and haemorrhage is difficult to control because the myocardium is thin and friable and the atrial pressures are abnormally high. Damage to coronary vessels is possible because they are not easy to identify and may be punctured by spicules of calcium. Myocardial failure is common because the muscle is fibrosed and thin, and dysrhythmias are sometimes a serious problem while the heart is displaced or distorted during dissection.

The induction of anaesthesia and initiation of controlled ventilation are less hazardous than in patients with cardiac tamponade and small doses of thiopentone can be used safely. The *operative* hazards are of much greater importance and these patients require continuous, detailed monitoring: ECG, intra-arterial recording of blood pressure, central venous pressure and urinary output. A period of artificial ventilation is generally necessary post-operatively, and a nasogastric tube should therefore be introduced before the patient leaves the theatre. Pharmacological support of the circulation may be needed, details of which can be found in Chapter 6.

INSERTION OF PACEMAKERS

Temporary pacing of the heart can be established using a transvenous, intraventricular wire attached to an external pacemaker. If permanent support is needed, a small battery-operated device is implanted in the tissues and is connected to the ventricle, either by electrodes attached to the surface of the heart, or using a transvenous wire. The wire reaches the right ventricle at one end while the other end is brought out subcutaneously to the battery. The transvenous system can be implanted under local anaesthesia, but general anaesthesia is required if electrodes are to be sewn onto the epicardium. The heart is generally approached from below, and the pacemaker is inserted into the anterior abdominal wall within the rectus sheath. In this site, even changing the pacemaker usually requires general anaesthesia.

A fixed rate pacemaker is satisfactory for most patients with long-standing complete heart block. Those with intermittent heart block require a unit which is suppressed if spontaneous ventricular beats occur regularly, but which initiates a new impulse if there is more than a predetermined delay before the next spontaneous beat. A few patients are supplied with a device which simulates normal sinus rhythm (Fig. 5.9). Spontaneous atrial systole triggers the pacemaker to initiate an impulse which then immediately provokes ventricular contraction. This enables the heart rate to change in response to physiological demands. Most implanted units require regular replacement, generally after about 3 years; external testing can indicate when this is necessary before irregularities of pacing occur.

Many of the patients are elderly, and the hazards of anaesthesia in old age are added to those associated with the procedure; episodes of circulatory failure are poorly tolerated and renal function in particular is often defective.

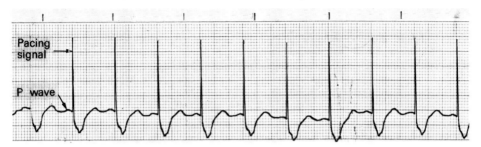

Figure 5.9 Cardiac pacing with an 'Atricor'. The P wave is followed by a high voltage signal from the pacing unit and this in turn is followed immediately by the QRS complex.

When complete heart block is present, the cardiac output can only change if the stroke volume alters; any reduction in ventricular filling or myocardial contractility must inevitably lower the output. If this causes hypotension and myocardial ischaemia, asystole or ventricular fibrillation may follow. The risk of cardiac standstill during induction of anaesthesia by any technique is so great that a temporary pacing wire should be inserted preoperatively in virtually all patients, certainly all those with symptomatic heart block of recent onset. Patients with long-standing heart block who only experience symptoms on exertion can, if necessary, be managed without, but isoprenaline should always be readily available in case the heart rate slows even further.

Anaesthetic management

The temporary wire is introduced through an antecubital, subclavian or internal jugular vein, and its tip can be dislodged from the ventricle by abduction of the arm, especially if the antecubital or subclavian routes have been chosen. Particular care must be taken to prevent disturbance while moving the patient from bed to operating table and ECG monitoring should continue throughout the period of temporary pacing, transfer to the theatre and the subsequent operation.

Atropine premedication is generally given but rarely causes significant changes in rate unless the heart block is intermittent. Anaesthesia can be induced with thiopentone and continued with nitrous oxide, provided satisfactory pacing has been established in those who need it (see above). Large doses of long-acting relaxants should be avoided because the operation is sometimes completed quickly if only the pacemaker unit requires changing.

A good intravenous infusion must always be established, even if only a change of pacemaker is anticipated. The integrity of the electrodes and the adequacy of their contact with the myocardium can only be confirmed when the pacemaker has been exposed, and it is sometimes necessary to change the electrodes as well as the unit; the myocardium can be torn at this stage and the massive haemorrhage which follows is difficult to control if access to the heart is poor.

Surgical diathermy can precipitate ventricular fibrillation in patients using a cardiac pacemaker and may also influence the rate of discharge of the pacing signal. It is preferable to avoid diathermy completely, but if an external pacemaker is in use and pacing can be discontinued without detriment to the circulation, the pacemaker must be switched off **and disconnected** before diathermy can be permitted. Once the permanent unit is in place, diathermy should not be used at all.

An internal pacemaker is either a unipolar or bipolar device. With the former, the circuit is complete when the metal surface of the unit (ground plate) is in contact with the patient's tissues, whereas with a bipolar system the circuit is formed through two electrodes attached to the myocardium. Once the electrodes are in place, the threshold voltage which just initiates ventricular systole is measured. When a bipolar system is being tested, first one and then the other lead is used as the active electrode. If the spontaneous ventricular rate is so slow that the cardiac output is inadequate without pacing, a very careful watch must be kept at this stage to ensure that a signal from either the temporary intravenous wire or the epicardial electrode is delivered with minimal interruption. Once satisfactory placement of the leads has been demonstrated, they are joined to the permanent unit and sealed in place. Temporary pacing can then be discontinued, but ECG monitoring must continue for at least 24 hours to confirm that the permanent system is working satisfactorily.

CARDIOVERSION

Synchronous DC defibrillation is used to convert a supraventricular dysrhythmia to sinus rhythm. Transitory asystole results from the passage of the current and, if successful, the sino-atrial node will initiate subsequent beats. The procedure can be undertaken electively (e.g. to convert atrial fibrillation to sinus rhythm in selected patients), but it may also be needed as an emergency to control life-threatening dysrhythmias. General anaesthesia is required unless the patient is *in extremis* because passage of the current causes a violent contraction of pectoral, intercostal and abdominal muscles and is therefore painful. A single dose of intravenous diazepam, methohexitone or 'Althesin' provides anaesthesia of sufficient duration if the first attempt at defibrillation is successful; it must also be possible to continue anaesthesia if necessary, for example with nitrous oxide and oxygen, and either halothane or increments of the intravenous agent used for induction. Premedication is often regarded as unnecessary or even undesirable, but it has been suggested that a vagolytic increases the success of the manœuvre.

Ventricular fibrillation is occasionally precipitated by cardioversion, and facilities for resuscitation must be readily available. It is wise to establish an intravenous route and ensure that this is adequately secured so that it cannot be displaced during defibrillation when manual restraint of the patient is impossible.

REFERENCES

The references quoted on the following topics apply to anaesthesia for both closed cardiac surgery and open heart procedures:
  General principles
  Muscle relaxants and their reversal

Effects of controlled ventilation

Humidification of the respiratory tract

References dealing with the effects of general anaesthetic agents and techniques, and those covering 'monitoring' during cardiac surgery are detailed at the end of Chapter 6.

GENERAL PRINCIPLES OF ANAESTHESIA FOR CARDIAC SURGERY

CULLEN D. J. (1974) Interpretation of blood pressure measurements in anesthesia. *Anesthesiology* **40**, 6.

DALTON B. (1972) Anesthesia for cardiac surgery (a letter of enquiry). *Anesthesiology* **36**, 522.

GILSTON A. (1971) Anaesthesia for cardiac surgery. *British Journal of Anaesthesia* **43**, 217.

HOWITT G. (1971) The pharmacology of the normal and diseased heart in relation to cardiac surgery. *British Journal of Anaesthesia* **43**, 261.

KELMAN G. R. (1971) Interpretation of central venous pressure measurements. *Anaesthesia* **26**, 209.

MOFFITT E. A., TARHAN S. & LUNDBORG R. O. (1968) Anesthesia for cardiac surgery: principles and practice. *Anesthesiology* **29**, 1181.

RUSSELL W. J. (1974) Central venous pressure in clinical use. *Part II of Central Venous Pressure: its clinical use and role in cardiovascular dynamics*. Butterworth, London.

MUSCLE RELAXANTS AND THEIR REVERSAL

COLEMAN A. J., DOWNING J. W., LEARY W. P., MOYES D. G. & STYLES M. (1972) The immediate cardiovascular effects of pancuronium, alcuronium and tubocurarine in man. *Anaesthesia* **27**, 415.

DUKE P. C., FUNG A. & GARTNER J. (1975) The myocardial effect of pancuronium. *Canadian Anaesthetists' Society Journal* **22**, 680.

HARRISON G. A. (1972) The cardiovascular effects and some relaxant properties of four relaxants in patients about to undergo cardiac surgery. *British Journal of Anaesthesia* **44**, 485.

SALEM M. R., YLAGAN L. B., ANGEL J. J., VEDAM V. S. & COLLINS V. J. (1970) Reversal of curarization with atropine-neostigmine mixture in patients with congenital cardiac disease. *British Journal of Anaesthesia* **42**, 991.

EFFECTS OF CONTROLLED VENTILATION

ADAMS A. P., ECONOMIDES A. P., FINLAY W. E. I. & SYKES M. K. (1970) The effects of variations of inspiratory flow waveform on cardiorespiratory function during controlled ventilation in normo-, hypo- and hypervolaemic dogs. *British Journal of Anaesthesia* **42**, 818.

BLACKBURN J. P., CONWAY C. M., LEIGH J. M., LINDOP M. J. & REITAN J. A. (1972) P_aCO_2 and the pre-ejection period: the P_aCO_2/inotropy response curve. *Anesthesiology* **37**, 268.

FOËX P. & PRYS-ROBERTS C. (1975) Effect of CO_2 on myocardial contractility and aortic input impedance during anaesthesia. *British Journal of Anaesthesia* **47**, 669.

PRYS-ROBERTS C., KELMAN G. R., GREENBAUM R. & ROBINSON R. H. (1967) Circulatory influences of artificial ventilation during nitrous oxide anaesthesia in man II. Results: the relative influence of mean intrathoracic pressure and arterial carbon dioxide tension. *British Journal of Anaesthesia* **39**, 533.

QVIST J., PONTOPPIDAN H., WILSON R. S., LOWENSTEIN E. & LAVER M. B. (1975) Hemodynamic responses to mechanical ventilation with PEEP: the effect of hypervolemia. *Anesthesiology* **42**, 45.

SEED R. F., SYKES M. K. & FINLAY W. E. L. (1970) Effect of variations in end-expiratory pressure on cardiorespiratory function before and after open heart surgery. *British Journal of Anaesthesia* **42**, 488.

TRICHET B., FALKE K., TOGUT A. & LAVER M. B. (1975) The effect of pre-existing pulmonary vascular disease on the response to mechanical ventilation with PEEP following open heart surgery. *Anesthesiology* **42**, 56.

VANCE J. P., BROWN D. M. & SMITH G. (1973) The effects of hypocapnia on myocardial blood flow and metabolism. *British Journal of Anaesthesia* **45**, 455.

HUMIDIFICATION OF THE RESPIRATORY TRACT

BOYS J. E. & HOWELLS T. H. (1972) Humidification in anaesthesia: a review of the present situation. *British Journal of Anaesthesia* **44**, 879.

CHALON J., LOEW D. A. Y. & MALEBRANCHE J. (1972) Effects of dry anesthetic gases on tracheobronchial ciliated epithelium. *Anesthesiology* **37**, 338.

FORBES A. R. (1973) Humidification and mucus flow in the intubated trachea. *British Journal of Anaesthesia* **45**, 874.

SHANKS C. A. (1974) Humidification and loss of body heat during anaesthesia II: effects in surgical patients. *British Journal of Anaesthesia* **46**, 863.

MITAL VALVOTOMY

FRASER K., TURNER M. A. & SUGDEN B. A. (1976) Closed mitral valvotomy. *British Medical Journal* **3**, 352.

Leading Article (1970) When to operate on the rheumatic mitral valve. *Lancet* **1**, 279.

SURGERY OF THE THORACIC AORTA

BENNETT E. J. & DALAL F. Y. (1974) Hypotensive anaesthesia for coarctation. A method of prevention of postoperative hypertension. *Anaesthesia* **29**, 269.

DALAL F. Y., BENNETT E. J., SALEM M. R. & EL-ETR A. A. (1974) Anaesthesia for coarctation. A new classification for rational anaesthetic management. *Anaesthesia* **29**, 704.

GOODALL McC. & SCALY W. C. (1969) Increased sympathetic nerve activity following resection of coarctation of the thoracic aorta. *Circulation* **39**, 345.

SABAWALA P. B., STRONG J. J. & KEATS A. S. (1970) Surgery of the aorta and its branches. *Anesthesiology* **33**, 229.

SLATER E. E. & DESANCTIS R. W. (1976) The clinical recognition of dissecting aortic aneurysm. *American Journal of Medicine* **60**, 625.

PERICARDIAL DISEASE

GABE I. T., MASON D. T., GAULT J. H., ROSS J. Jr., ZELIS R., MILLS C. J., BRAUNWALD E. & SHILLINGFORD J. P. (1970) Effect of respiration on venous return and stroke volume in cardiac tamponade. *British Heart Journal* **32**, 592.

SHARP J. T., BUNNELL I. L., HOLLAND J. F., GRIFFITH G. T. & GREENE D. G. (1960) Hemodynamics during induced cardiac tamponade in man. *American Journal of Medicine* **29**, 640.

CARDIAC PACING

ORLAND H. J. & JONES D. (1975) Cardiac pacemaker induced ventricular fibrillation during surgical diathermy. *Anaesthesia and Intensive Care* **3**, 321.

SCOTT D. L. (1970) Cardiac pacemakers as an anaesthetic problem. *Anaesthesia* **25**, 87.

SOWTON E., SPURRELL R. & ROY P. (1975) Clinical use of pacemakers in the treatment of conduction disturbances. *Advances in Cardiology* **14**, 266.

CARDIOVERSION

ORKO R. (1974) Anaesthesia for cardioversion: thiopentone with and without atropine premedication. *British Journal of Anaesthesia* **46**, 947.

ORKO R. (1976) Anaesthesia for cardioversion: a comparison of diazepam, thiopentone and propanidid. *British Journal of Anaesthesia* **48**, 257.

SOMERS K., GUNSTONE R. F., PATEL A. K. & D'ARBELA P. G. (1971) Intravenous diazepam for direct current cardioversion. *British Medical Journal* **4**, 13.

CHAPTER 6

ANAESTHESIA FOR OPEN HEART SURGERY

The term 'open heart surgery' embraces all those procedures in which the operative requirements preclude maintenance of an effective circulation by the heart. During this period, some form of extracorporeal support is required, and the heart can then be opened widely and accurate surgery carried out under direct vision in a virtually bloodless field. There has been a rapid expansion during the last two decades in the scope of surgical procedures which are feasible under these conditions; even grossly disabled patients can now be restored to near normal health, provided the haemodynamic abnormality can be corrected. It is for this reason that disturbances which greatly increase the risks of general anaesthesia can never be regarded as a contraindication to operation. In general, the severity of the preoperative condition and the magnitude of the procedure combine to render open heart surgery more

hazardous than the majority of closed procedures. Good preoperative preparation may lessen disability, but it is often necessary to proceed in patients
with little functional reserve in one or more vital system (Fig. 6.1).

CHOICE OF ANAESTHETIC TECHNIQUE

Induction and maintenance

The arguments in favour of generous premedication whenever possible have
been set out in Chapter 3; exceptions to this rule are dealt with individually.
Similarly, the general principles governing the management of anaesthesia
during cardiac surgery have been discussed in Chapter 5 but there are two
additional features which warrant particular consideration during open heart
surgery. The first is the desirability of maintaining a moderate degree of peripheral vasodilatation and the second is the probable necessity for a period
of ventilatory support postoperatively.

Peripheral vasoconstriction is a consequence of severe cardiac failure, of
induced hypothermia and of the procedure of cardiopulmonary bypass itself.
Although the systemic vascular resistance commonly falls at the onset of bypass when haemodilution causes an abrupt reduction in blood viscosity, there

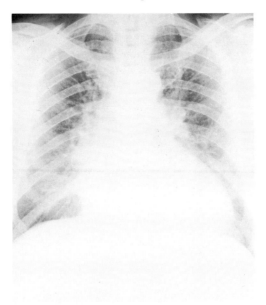

Figure 6.1 Uncontrolled left ventricular failure before open heart surgery: male
aged 72 years with hypertension, ischaemic heart disease, mitral regurgitation and
a left ventricular aneurysm. The left atrial pressure was recorded during operation
as 115/40 mm Hg (15.3/5·3 kPa) relative to the mix-axillary line.

is a subsequent gradual increase in arteriolar tone, possibly related to elevation of the arterial oxygen tension, hypocapnia or rising levels of circulating catecholamines. As a result, perfusion of capillary beds is impaired and metabolic acidosis develops, even though the flow rate from the oxygenator and the mean arterial blood pressure are high. If peripheral vasoconstriction persists when a spontaneous heart beat is restored, cardiac work is expended on the generation of pressure rather than flow, and the cardiac output is often low in spite of a relatively normal systolic blood pressure. Poor tissue perfusion continues and myocardial function deteriorates as the metabolic acidosis becomes more severe.

Some degree of arteriolar vasodilatation is desirable, therefore, although the presence of warm, pink skin should not be taken to indicate that all the vascular beds are well perfused. It must also be remembered that adequate flow through the microcirculation depends upon an essential minimum head of pressure, the 'critical closing pressure'. This can still be exceeded when the aortic blood pressure is relatively low, provided there is no arterial disease limiting the transmission of pressure to the vessels beyond. This proviso does not always apply in some tissue beds (e.g. the brain or coronary circulation), and in such circumstances, ischaemic damage can be caused if the mean aortic pressure is low because a high flow is being delivered against a relatively low resistance, most of the blood being distributed to tissue beds of relatively little importance. The hazard is even greater if the peripheral resistance is lowered by drugs when overall flow is poor; unless the reduction in afterload permits an increase in stroke volume, the perfusion of vital organs may fall while blood flow to non-essential tissues increases.

Peripheral vasoconstriction is often a feature of general anaesthesia with thiopentone, nitrous oxide, oxygen, muscle relaxants and controlled ventilation. However, the technique is simple and reliable, and vasoconstriction can be minimised by the liberal use of opiate analgesics and the avoidance of hypocapnia. Drugs with specific, short-acting vasodilator properties (e.g. phentolamine) can always be added if required, particularly during cardiopulmonary bypass.

There is a preference in some centres for anaesthetic agents which promote vasodilatation from the outset. The neuroleptic combination droperidol and fentanyl has α-adrenergic blocking properties and causes very little myocardial depression. Anaesthesia can be induced gradually using incremental doses of droperidol (2·5–5 mg) and fentanyl (0·125–0·25 mg) to a total dose of approximately 100 μg/kg of droperidol and 10 μg/kg of fentanyl; although rather time-consuming, induction is pleasant and the patient generally remains calm. Peripheral perfusion is good as judged by skin blood flow and urine output, and the incidence of dysrhythmias is said to be low because of the anti-adrenergic properties of droperidol and the profound analgesic effect of fentanyl. Undesirable hypotension is rare unless excessive increments

of droperidol are given; occasionally patients develop muscular rigidity following intravenous fentanyl but this can always be controlled with relaxants.

An alternative technique which promotes peripheral vasodilatation consists of anaesthesia with large doses of intravenous morphine sulphate (1–
5 mg/kg). Hypotension is unusual provided the rate of injection does not
exceed 5 mg/minute and crystalloid solutions are infused generously, myocardial function is not impaired and myocardial oxygen consumption probably falls. Ventilation can often be controlled without muscle relaxants, and
the prolonged respiratory depression is regarded as desirable because of the
continued need for controlled ventilation in the postoperative period. Nitrous
oxide is usually avoided because some myocardial depression can be demonstrated when nitrous oxide replaces oxygen during morphine anaesthesia, but
hypnosis and amnesia during surgery cannot be ensured in all patients given
unsupplemented intravenous morphine with oxygen. This method has
achieved some popularity in American centres but is not widely used in the
UK.

The choice of technique is probably of less importance than ensuring that
it is implemented smoothly. Coughing and straining cause hypoxia and elevation of the venous pressure while surgical stimulation in the presence of inadequate anaesthesia leads to dangerous hypertension and tachycardia. Both
hypoxia and hypercarbia are deleterious—rhythm disturbances may be provoked, myocardial function is depressed, the response to adrenergic stimulants is impaired, hyperkalaemia can develop and pulmonary vasoconstriction is inevitable. Hypocapnia ($P_a CO_2$ less than 4·0 kPa) is also undesirable
because it accentuates both peripheral and cerebral vasoconstriction and
lowers the cardiac output.

Ventilation

Open heart surgery is usually carried out through a sternal-splitting incision
and both pleural cavities remain intact. Interference with the movement of
the lungs is less common than during many closed cardiac procedures, but
sometimes the pleura is punctured or even opened widely; either a pneumo-
thorax or an accumulation of blood in the pleural space can then embarrass
ventilation.

The effects of artificial ventilation in patients with heart disease differ from
those seen in normal subjects. The interplay of haemodynamic and respiratory variables is complex and the net result within the individual depends
upon the nature and severity of pulmonary and cardiac pathology.

The majority of the haemodynamic effects of intermittent positive
pressure ventilation (IPPV) are attributable to an increase in intrathoracic
pressure. This lowers the filling pressure of the heart, transfers part of the
pulmonary blood volume into the systemic capacitance vessels and normally

causes a fall in cardiac output. The output returns to normal if the venous tone rises or if the intravascular volume is increased. When the heart is failing, the elevation of intrathoracic pressure during IPPV is relatively small by comparison with the ventricular filling pressures which are already high, the influence of changes in filling pressure on stroke volume is less than normal, and the blood volume is usually increased. The fall in cardiac output which accompanies IPPV is therefore less apparent as heart failure becomes more severe.

The pulmonary sequelae of heart disease (p. 12) interfere with efficient gas exchange. The alveolar–arterial oxygen tension gradient $[(A-a)DO_2]$ is generally elevated, even in the absence of a right to left intracardiac shunt, and the dead space:tidal volume ratio (V_D/V_T) is abnormally high. Positive pressure ventilation, particularly with a large tidal volume delivered at a slow rate, with an end-inspiratory pause, and possibly with a positive pressure during expiration, improves the distribution of inspired gas. Alveoli which fill slowly are recruited if inspiration is prolonged, previously atelectatic areas can be reinflated, and the generation of pulmonary oedema is impeded. This leads to a decrease in $(A-a)DO_2$, particularly if pulmonary blood flow to atelectatic areas has remained virtually normal.

IPPV also eliminates the work of breathing. This may be excessive if there is both pulmonary disease and a limited cardiac output with which to sustain the oxygen requirements of the respiratory muscles. The elimination of part of the systemic oxygen requirement redresses imbalance between oxygen demands and the limited oxygen supply available to the tissues; although the cardiac output may fall, the mixed venous oxygen content rises.

The rise in intrathoracic pressure which accompanies IPPV tends to increase the resistance to right ventricular ejection and might therefore be considered undesirable when pulmonary hypertension is present. However, the increase in pulmonary vascular resistance caused by IPPV is trivial by comparison with the vascular resistance already present, and the effect is often more than offset by the reduction in right ventricular after-load which follows displacement of blood out of the lungs. At the same time, the work of breathing is eliminated and the preservation of normal arterial glood gas tensions prevents any increase in pulmonary vascular tone caused by hypoxia or hypercapnia.

The beneficial effects of positive pressure ventilation, and particularly those of positive end-expiratory pressure on gas exchange are less prominent in patients with pulmonary vascular disease than in those in whom the pulmonary vascular resistance is virtually normal. Ventilation to previously atelectatic areas may improve arterial oxygenation, but the effect will be minimal if pulmonary blood flow to the same territory is reduced because of pre-existing pulmonary vascular disease. At the same time, the arterial carbon dioxide tension will rise if the dead space/tidal volume ratio is increased by the application of positive end-expiratory pressure.

Two potentially undesirable effects of IPPV must also be considered. Factors which increase the resistance to blood flow through the lungs (or decrease the systemic vascular resistance) augment flow through a right to left intracardiac shunt and accentuate arterial hypoxaemia. A pattern of ventilation should be chosen for these patients which minimises the increase in intrathoracic pressure, but a negative pressure during expiration is not recommended because it favours alveolar collapse. Secondly, unnecessary hyperventilation decreases the arterial carbon dioxide tension and leads to a fall in cardiac output which is independent of changes in intrathoracic pressure.

It is customary to use mechanical rather than manual ventilation during surgery. The ventilator must be capable of generating pressures which are sufficient to inflate lungs of poor compliance and high airway resistance, and it is preferable to use a volume preset device so that changes in pulmonary characteristics will have only minimal effect on alveolar ventilation. A humidifier should be incorporated into the circuit because anaesthesia is sometimes prolonged and generally precedes a further period of mechanical ventilation.

MONITORING

Circulation

Electrocardiograph   The ECG is monitored routinely throughout all open heart surgery. Subcutaneous needle electrodes are more reliable than most surface electrodes because neither sweat nor blood spilled onto the skin cause electrical interference.

Arterial blood pressure   Sphygmomanometry is rarely satisfactory because moment to moment changes in pressure are common and intermittent recording provides insufficient information. In addition, peripheral pulses are absent during the virtually non-pulsatile perfusion of cardiopulmonary bypass and they may be imperceptible when vasoconstriction is intense. It is preferable to monitor the pressure continuously using an indwelling radial arterial cannula; with experience, this can be introduced percutaneously in virtually every case, including infants and children. The cannula requires some rigidity to prevent the tip buckling as it passes through the arterial wall, and Teflon cannulae are preferable to those made from polypropylene because thrombus forms less readily on the surface. Damage to surrounding tissues is rare unless the cannula is flushed inadvertently with irritant or sclerosing solutions and there is a lower incidence of postoperative obliteration of the pulse if a narrow, parallel-sided cannula is used, as distinct from one which is tapered throughout its length from hub to tip. Loss of the radial pulse occurs in some cases but even complete occlusion of the artery does not cause ischaemia of the hand if the ulnar artery is present and patent. The adequacy of the blood supply which can be derived through the ulnar artery can be ascertained before cannulation in a number of ways. One of the most simple is to apply digital pressure to the radial artery at the wrist. Pulsation in the radial artery distal to the site of compression, which can only be eliminated by simultaneous compression of the ulnar artery, indicates that there is a satisfactory flow through the palmar arch system via the ulnar artery.

The brachial, ulnar or femoral vessels are sometimes used if radial arterial puncture is unsuccessful. This entails a greater risk of ischaemia in tissues distal to the site of cannulation, and it is probably wiser to abandon percutaneous cannulation; a cut-down exposes the radial artery which can generally be cannulated directly even when it is impalpable.

After the cannula has been introduced, it should be flushed periodically with *small* (0·5 ml) increments of heparinised Ringer-lactate solution which has a more physiological pH than normal saline. If larger volumes are injected vigorously through the arterial line, there is a higher incidence of local ischaemic damage, and air bubbles or thrombi can be flushed in a retrograde direction into other branches of the subclavian artery.

The cannula is connected to a suitable transducer so that the blood pressure can be displayed continuously and permanent recordings made when necessary. Persistent damping of the pressure waveform is sometimes troublesome even when the system is free from leaks or trapped air bubbles. Papaverine (10–40 mg) diluted in 2–5 ml of Ringer-lactate solution can be injected slowly through the arterial line to promote local vasodilatation and so preserve accurate pressure monitoring.

Central venous and left atrial pressures Both the superior and inferior vena caval pressures must be monitored during bypass because either vessel may be obstructed by the introduction of cannulae which drain blood from the heart to the extracorporeal apparatus. In a few cases, drainage is undertaken with only a single right atrial cannula rather than two caval cannulae, and then only one venous pressure need be monitored. It is possible to place intravenous catheters percutaneously in both cavae, either before or after the induction of anaesthesia. The superior vena cava is approached via the internal jugular, subclavian, or antecubital veins. The external jugular vein is less satisfactory because the tip of the cannula can rarely be advanced beyond the clavicle and can easily be obstructed by movement of the head postoperatively. Extravasation into the tissues around deeply situated veins cannot be detected easily, and local damage may occur if irritant drugs are injected; unrecognised and subsequently fatal haemorrhage has been reported following superior caval cannulation via the vessels of the head and neck. A cannula of adequate length (at least 10 cm for an adult) must be used for the internal jugular or subclavian veins to ensure that its tip is within the lumen of the vessel, some distance beyond the puncture site. However, a catheter more than 15 cm long may be caught in the superior caval snare during bypass. Correct placement should be confirmed immediately after the cannula has been inserted: the transfusion bottle is lowered to below table height while the intravenous tubing control remains widely open. Blood will flow back freely into the tubing if the tip of the cannula is intravascular.

The inferior vena caval pressure can be monitored by cannulation of the femoral veins although this is sometimes considered undesirable because of the risks of thrombosis or sepsis, or because access to the groin is needed surgically. As an alternative, a 'Redding cannula', which has a pressure-monitoring channel fused to its wall, can be used to drain the inferior cava during bypass. If femoral vein cannulation is not carried out preoperatively, some anaesthetists elect to establish a second upper limb infusion so that blood replacement and venous pressure monitoring can be carried out independently. This also facilitates the administration of supportive drugs by infusion in the postoperative period. In the unusual event of central venous cannulation proving impossible, surgery can be started with only a peripheral infusion in place; a long cannula can then be introduced at operation into the right atrium or innominate vein and brought out through the chest wall for postoperative use.

A similar technique is used to establish left atrial pressure monitoring. A fine catheter is introduced either directly into the left atrium or through a pulmonary vein, and it too is brought out through the chest wall. Alternatively, the left atrial line is inserted via the right atrium and interatrial septum. Care must be taken to ensure that these lines are not snared in sutures while the chest is being closed, and gentle traction should be sufficient to remove them postoperatively. Haemorrhage is rare following their withdrawal, but it is wise to remove the monitoring lines before the chest drainage tubes.

Embolism, particularly of air, is a special hazard of left atrial pressure monitoring. Particular care must be taken to avoid the introduction of air when the cannula is connected to a pressure transducer, and a blocked line should never be flushed vigorously for fear of displacing clot into the systemic circulation. An intravenous cannula is equally hazardous in patients with a right to left shunt. All intravenous tubing and the galleries of taps on these lines should be filled very carefully to eliminate trapped air bubbles.

All pressure measurements must be referred to a consistent zero level— commonly either the sternal angle or the mid-axillary line. Whichever is chosen, it must be possible to adjust the height of the transducers when the height of the operating table is altered during surgery.

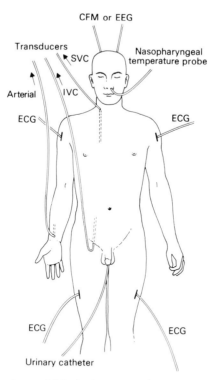

Figure 6.2 Monitoring established prior to open heart surgery. A catheter introduced at operation will be used to monitor left atrial pressure postoperatively.

The *cardiac output* is sometimes monitored routinely using either a dye or thermal dilution technique, or a retractable electromagnetic flow probe which is secured around the aorta with a slip stitch. Once this stitch is released, the probe can be removed through the chest wall when the need for monitoring has passed.

Gas exchange and acid-base balance

Arterial blood can be sampled easily and repeatedly through the radial arterial cannula and pressure-monitoring system. Measurements are generally made in apparatus which is maintained at a temperature of 37°C, and correction factors may need to be applied if the patient's body temperature deviates significantly from this value; nomograms are available for this purpose (p. 152). The frequency with which gas tensions and pH should be estimated varies from case to case. Routine analysis is not always performed during straightforward surgery undertaken by experienced teams, but facilities for the investigation must always be readily available.

Biochemical and haematological monitoring

Potassium   Changes in electrolyte composition are common during cardio-pulmonary bypass, fluctuations in the plasma potassium concentration being of the greatest importance. Patients who have been treated intensively with diuretics preoperatively may be potassium depleted (p. 19), while the potassium concentration during operation is influenced by many factors such as dilution with the priming fluid in the extracorporeal circuit, changes in acid–base balance, the administration of potassium salts, and above all, by urinary loss if (as commonly occurs) a massive diuresis is established during perfusion.

Potassium is predominantly an intracellular ion and the margins of safety for the extracellular concentration are small, too little causing an increase in ventricular excitability and too much resulting in myocardial depression. Generous replacement is often required (e.g. 30–150 mmol during the course of operation), and facilities for the rapid estimation of plasma potassium are as necessary as those for pH and blood gas monitoring.

Haematocrit   At the present time, little or no blood is added to the priming volume in the extracorporeal circuit (p. 143) for surgery in adult patients, and serial measurements of haematocrit are used to assess the degree of haemodilution which occurs when this prime is mixed with the patient's blood. Monitoring the haematocrit is of particular importance in patients with cyanotic congenital heart disease and secondary polycythaemia because it is often desirable to achieve a sustained reduction in red cell concentration.

Free haemoglobin   Serial measurements of the concentration of free haemoglobin are sometimes requested to document the extent of haemolysis and blood damage, most of which occurs in the suction apparatus which returns blood from the operating field to the oxygenator.

Blood coagulation   Whole body heparinisation is necessary during cardio-pulmonary bypass, and a number of tests have been advocated for the control of both the dose of heparin and its reversal with protamine sulphate. These include the whole blood coagulation time, the thrombin time, the activated partial thromboplastin time and the blood activated recalcification time. Unfortunately, several of them are too insensitive for monitoring clinically important degrees of heparinisation, and both heparin and protamine are often prescribed empirically. Recently, an automated method for determining the coagulation time, and the 'BART' test, a modification of the whole blood-activated recalcification time, have been recommended for speedy and reliable evaluation of heparin activity during surgery.

The platelet count falls dramatically during bypass and a number of intrinsic coagulation factors may be diluted or destroyed (p. 185). Specific tests can be used to determine the nature of coagulation defects but they are often time-consuming, difficult to interpret, and are rarely undertaken as a routine.

Urine output

In the absence of renal disease, the urine output is a sensitive index of the adequacy of tissue perfusion. In addition, knowledge of its volume and composition facilitates fluid and electrolyte replacement. A diuresis commonly occurs during bypass because large volumes of non-colloidal fluids are used in the oxygenator; renal perfusion improves when the extracorporeal system replaces the failing heart, and the reduction in haematocrit leads to an increase in renal plasma flow.

A catheter is introduced with full aseptic precautions immediately before operation. It is connected to a graduated drainage system so that urine output can be measured accurately at short intervals and aliquots can be removed for the determination of urinary electrolyte concentrations, particularly potassium. The catheter remains in place postoperatively until the need for frequent assessment has passed and the patient is awake and well enough to control micturition.

Temperature

Hypothermia is a common feature of open heart surgery. It may be induced electively (p. 150) to decrease tissue oxygen requirements or it may occur spontaneously because temperature regulation is impaired by prolonged anaesthesia, circulatory failure, heat loss from the widely opened thoracic incision, or the transfusion of cold blood. Cooling rarely occurs uniformly, even when active steps are taken to promote vasodilatation and good tissue perfusion, and it may be necessary to record temperature in several sites. The mid-oesophagus and nasopharynx are commonly chosen because temperatures here are considered to reflect myocardial and cerebral temperature respectively. The adequacy of peripheral perfusion can be assessed by monitoring the difference between the 'core' or central temperature (rectum, oesophagus or nasopharynx) and a peripheral site (toe or somatic muscle). Calibrated thermocouples mounted in needles or flexible probes are used according to site. Care is needed if temperature probes are introduced through the nose because minor trauma to the mucosa sometimes causes troublesome haemorrhage when the patient is subsequently heparinised.

Cerebral function

Brain damage can complicate cardiac surgery, either because there has been an episode of cardiac arrest or prolonged circulatory failure, or because embolism or inadequate perfusion have complicated the surgical repair and

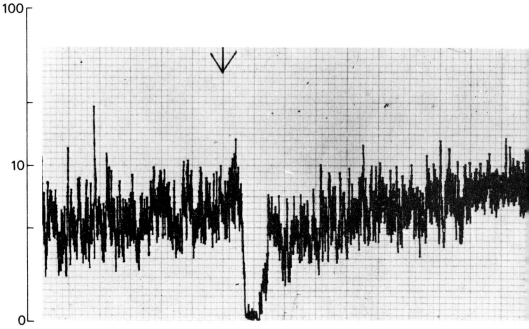

Figure 6.3 Cerebral function during cardiopulmonary bypass recorded on the Cerebral Function Monitor (paper speed 6 mm min^{-1}). The circulation was interrupted briefly at the arrow causing a transitory absence of cerebral activity; the patient regained consciousness uneventfully.

bypass procedure. Patients vary in the degree to which they can tolerate haemodynamic disturbances, and monitoring the electroencephalograph (EEG) gives some indication of the adequacy of cerebral function. Only cortical disturbances can be detected, and focal lesions may be inapparent if they occur far away from the site of a monitoring electrode. Conventional EEG monitoring is cumbersome, and recording during surgery is difficult because of electrical interference, particularly from diathermy apparatus. Interpretation is also difficult unless expert advice is available. A heavily filtered two-channel EEG recorded slowly ('Cerebral Function Monitor', Devices Ltd), provides useful information about the integrity of the cerebral cortex and the timing of disturbances. The signal is derived from two intradermal platinum needle electrodes inserted in the parietal region on either side of the midline, approximately 5 cm apart and a little behind the level of a line joining the external auditory meati. The ouput appears as a broad band of electrical activity, and disturbances are indicated by an alteration in the mean level or amplitude of the tracing (Fig. 6.3).

Patient safety

The complex monitoring required during open heart surgery generally entails the use of several independent instruments. Should the performance of any one of these be faulty, the patient may suffer electrical burns or even electrocution. Ideally, all monitoring apparatus should be 'floating' and therefore isolated from the mains. Alternatively, it should be locked to a common earth to which the patient is also attached through the indifferent electrode of the diathermy apparatus. Isolating transformers are commonly present in current electromedical apparatus and some also include warning devices which are operated by faults in the isolation circuit.

MANAGEMENT DURING CARDIOPULMONARY BYPASS

A detailed account of cardiopulmonary bypass is included in Chapter 8, but in brief the technique entails drainage of blood by gravity from the superior and inferior venae cavae into an oxygenator where gas exchange takes place. Blood is pumped back either to the ascending aorta or occasionally to the femoral artery. Flow is retrograde, towards the heart, but blood cannot enter the left ventricle unless the aortic valve is incompetent and so a head of pressure is generated in the aorta which is sufficient to disperse the flow throughout the systemic arterial system. If the aortic valve is incompetent or is the site of surgery, obstruction to the retrograde flow of blood in the aorta is provided by an aortic cross-clamp. This excludes the coronary vessels from the perfusion system and may necessitate the provision of a separate arterial supply to them. Suckers are used to return intracardiac blood to the oxygenator, and a separate drainage tube, the left ventricular vent, is often needed to prevent overdistension of the left heart (Fig. 6.4).

Until snares placed round the cavae are tightened, so occluding the vessel against its contained cannula, some blood can still enter the right atrium around the outside of the cannulae. Provided the heart is beating, this blood flows through the lungs in the usual way and is ejected into the systemic circulation against the perfusion pressure from the extracorporeal apparatus. Pressure transients are then seen in time with the heart beat, superimposed

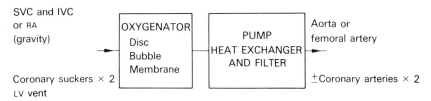

Figure 6.4 Simplified diagram to illustrate the principles of cardiopulmonary bypass.

on the perfusion pressure maintained by the pump. This condition is known
as partial cardiopulmonary bypass.

Anaesthetic management during cardiopulmonary bypass can be considered under the following headings:

1   Control of coagulation.
2   Maintenance of unconsciousness.
3   Control of ventilation.
4   Induction of elective cardiac arrest.
5   Restoration of the heart beat.
6   Termination of perfusion.
7   Myocardial support.

Control of coagulation

It is essential for blood to be completely incoagulable during perfusion. If
it is not, contact with the foreign surfaces of the apparatus initiates coagulation which can either obstruct the circuit or cause defibrination and
intractable postperfusion haemorrhage. These hazards are eliminated by
maintaining full heparinisation throughout perfusion. However, individual
requirements for heparin vary, and few of the tests used for controlling the
dose are entirely satisfactory (p. 84). It is customary therefore to use large
doses which ensure that heparin is always present in excess.

Mucous heparin is given intravenously just before the heart is cannulated;
multidose vials contain preservative and should not be used. The dose is usually calculated according to the body weight (3 mg/kg), but is sometimes determined on the basis of surface area (90 mg/m^2). An interval of at least 3
minutes should elapse between the administration of heparin and the introduction of cannulae. This allows the drug to circulate freely, even if the heart
is greatly enlarged or the circulation time is prolonged. Adequate mixing of
the heparin is particularly essential if the arterial return enters the femoral
artery. Cannulation excludes the rest of the limb from the circulation, and
distal thrombosis occurs unless the blood is incoagulable.

Heparin is metabolised rapidly by some patients, and unless accurate
monitoring of the degree of anticoagulation is available, a further dose (0·5 mg/
kg) should be given if more than 30 minutes elapse between the initial dose
of heparin and the onset of bypass. Additional increments are necessary at
30 to 60-minute intervals during perfusion but are generally injected directly
into the extracorporeal apparatus.

Maintenance of unconsciousness

There are conflicting factors which influence the level of anaesthesia at the
onset of bypass. Anaesthetic drugs are diluted in the priming volume of the
extracorporeal circuit and inhalational agents can be excreted into the gas

mixture in the oxygenator. At the same time, cerebral metabolism is depressed by the perfusion itself, perhaps because of ischaemic or embolic damage, or because a pulsatile arterial pressure waveform is lost. Hypothermia augments this depression of cerebral metabolism. In general, anaesthesia tends to lighten during partial bypass, but this is unlikely once the caval snares have been tightened and the aorta cross-clamped.

An increment of thiopentone, droperidol, or a narcotic analgesic is commonly given at the onset of perfusion and can be injected intravenously or added to the oxygenator. It is followed by an additional dose of muscle relaxant which prevents the return of spontaneous ventilation when IPPV is discontinued (see below). Further doses of relaxant may be required subsequently if there is a large diuresis, but extra sedation is not always necessary. Many of the physical signs of lightening anaesthesia are abolished by perfusion, but changes in pupillary size and lacrimation can still occur. They are rarely seen in spite of the small quantites of anaesthetic agents which are used; complaints of awareness during surgery are indefensible, but are no more common than during other procedures carried out under light anaesthesia. Low concentrations of halothane are sometimes added to the fresh gases supplied to the oxygenator, but some myocardial depression results and halothane is chemically incompatible with equipment containing polycarbonate resins.

Control of ventilation

Ventilation of the lungs is no longer required once full bypass has been established; it may even be disadvantageous because it disturbs the surgical field and causes movement of blood in and out of the open heart so producing a dangerous froth. During partial bypass, blood is being delivered from the left ventricle into the systemic circulation for as long as arterial pressure transients are visible in time with the heart beat. This blood should be oxygenated, and therefore artificial ventilation is required. The ventilatory volume and pattern are not altered, and normal arterial gas tensions will be maintained provided the gas mixture supplied to the oxygenator is of the correct composition (p. 145). As a general rule, IPPV is discontinued when pressure transients disappear from the arterial waveform. An important exception to this rule occurs when aortic cross-clamping is performed early while the heart is still beating. Until the heart has been opened, the left ventricle continues to supply the coronary arteries, and ventilation should be continued if possible to ensure that this blood is oxygenated.

It is sometimes suggested that a slight positive pressure in the lungs during the period of apnoea helps to prevent alveolar collapse. Ideally, the lungs should be distended with an inert gas. In practice, it is common to supply a minimal flow of oxygen although it could be argued that this is deleterious and may even augment alveolar collapse if there is any blood flowing through the lungs at all (e.g. from bronchial collaterals). One practical advantage of maintaining a slight positive pressure in the lungs is the presence of a distended anaesthetic bag which facilitates the detection of minimal respiratory movements.

A request is often made towards the end of the surgical procedure for gentle positive pressure ventilation. This helps to drive blood out of the pulmonary veins and clear both these and the left heart of any entrapped air. It should be carried out manually, and slight sustained positive pressure should be maintained while the closing stitches are placed in the left heart. Once the heart has been closed, artificial ventilation will no longer generate foam within the cardiac cavities, but it may still be disadvantageous if movement of the lungs encroaches on the surgical field. The time at which IPPV is restarted is dependent therefore on recognition of need (return of ejection from the heart, signified by pressure transients on the arterial waveform), and the absence of contraindication (residual open cardiac cavity, or surgery when pulmonary movement would be disturbing). A few breaths of sustained manual hyperinflation at the onset of IPPV help to re-expand atelectatic areas.

Elective cardiac arrest

Several operations can only be undertaken safely on a virtually motionless heart, and it may therefore be necessary to induce either ventricular fibrillation or asystole. Ventricular fibrillation can be induced by the passage of a

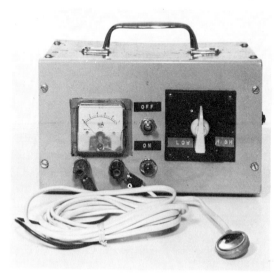

Figure 6.5 A fibrillator with its lead. The two surfaces of the electrode are separated by an insulating layer. One surface is placed in contact with the heart; the circuit is completed by contact of the other surface with the pericardial cavity.

small, low voltage, direct current through the heart (Fig. 6.5); asystole results from ischaemia (cross-clamping the aorta without coronary perfusion) or from perfusion of the heart with potassium-containing solutions. There are advantages and disadvantages to each method and the choice is generally governed by surgical preference.

Some myocardial damage is inflicted whichever technique is employed, but provided good coronary perfusion is ultimately restored, satisfactory function will generally return, even in a heart which has been ischaemic for so long that electrical silence has been reached. Selective hypothermia is sometimes used to diminish myocardial oxygen requirements when episodes of ischaemia are anticipated. Iced saline is infused into the pericardial sac and chambers of the heart, the flow being regulated to avoid flooding the surgical field. Alternatively, the fibrillating myocardium is perfused whenever possible, either by separate cannulation of the coronary ostia (p. 137) or by intermittently releasing the aortic cross-clamp when it is both safe and convenient to do so.

Restoration of the heart beat

If the heart has been beating throughout the operation, it may be possible to discontinue bypass as soon as surgery has been completed and the patient is warm. Electively induced ventricular fibrillation is likely to persist when the fibrillating electrode is removed, and the asystolic heart commonly returns to ventricular fibrillation when it is rewarmed and perfused. Occasionally, ventricular fibrillation reverts spontaneously to sinus rhythm, but more often electrical defibrillation is required.

Defibrillation   A DC shock of 25–100 Joules is used depending on the size of the heart and the ease with which the electrodes can be applied to its surface. It may be impossible or dangerous to free the ventricle when there are dense adhesions between the heart and pericardium, and then the electrodes cannot be placed so that the shock is delivered across the ventricular mass. Defibrillation may be successful if a larger shock is used, or alternatively it can be attempted using sterile external electrodes.

Defibrillation is often successful at the first attempt, provided the fibrillation is coarse and the electrodes can be applied satisfactorily.

If initial attempts at defibrillation are unsuccessful, the following questions should be asked:

1   Is the central temperature too low? Defibrillation is unlikely to succeed unless the core temperature is above 32°C.
2   Is the patient hypoxic or is there a respiratory or metabolic acidosis?
3   Is the plasma potassium concentration abnormal?
4   Is there a mechanical cause, e.g. unrecognised aortic incompetence? obstruction of a newly inserted prosthetic valve? distortion or damage to a coronary vessel? coronary air embolism?

5   Is there a fault in the defibrillator or its leads?

Subsequent management depends upon the answers to these questions, but, in general, two conditions can be recognised. The first is the presence of coarse ventricular fibrillation which may momentarily defibrillate to a coordinated rhythm, but then, almost instantly, reverts to fibrillation. Provided the treatable causes enumerated above have been eliminated, defibrillation can be attempted again after the administration of a bolus of lignocaine (1–2 mg/kg). Occasionally, verapamil (1·25–5 mg) is more effective. It is rarely safe to suppress ventricular excitability at this stage with β-adrenergic blocking drugs.

Myocardial tone must be improved if coarse ventricular fibrillation cannot be established. A prolonged period of cardiopulmonary bypass with good coronary perfusion is often effective. The heart is left undisturbed and overdistension is avoided by draining the left ventricle through the vent. Inotropic agents such as isoprenaline (5–20 μg), adrenaline (10–100 μg) or calcium chloride (0·5–2·5 mmol) can be given and glucagon or corticosteroids (p. 95) are used occasionally.

Management of other dysrhythmias   Sinus rhythm is not always resumed either when the heart beat returns spontaneously or following defibrillation. Some dysrhythmias can be tolerated without detriment to the performance of the heart, but others prevent the maintenance of an adequate circulation. An outline of their management is given below, but new measures are introduced frequently and may modify the choice of drug therapy.

Heart block   An infusion of isoprenaline (2–10 μg/min) increases the ventricular rate and sometimes decreases the degree of atrioventricular dissociation. Large doses are often required, and there is always a risk of sudden ventricular fibrillation because the drug also increases ventricular excitability. Alternatively, extreme bradycardia or asystole may follow if the infusion is interrupted. It is safer to institute electrical pacing if complete heart block is present. Epicardial wires are attached to the heart and are subsequently brought out through the chest wall. Ventricular contraction should follow a stimulus of between 0·5 and 2·0 volts from an external battery. Some units cannot provide an impulse more frequently than 100 times per minute, and if the ventricular rate exceeds this because isoprenaline is being given, the infusion should be slowed or stopped so that the pacemaker can 'capture' the ventricle and govern its subsequent rate of contraction.

A permanent pacing unit is not inserted unless heart block was present preoperatively. Temporary pacing wires are sometimes attached prophylactically; they can be used postoperatively if required, but are otherwise removed by gentle traction after a few days.

Corticosteroids are occasionally recommended to reduce inflammation around a recently damaged atrioventricular node or Bundle of His. There is little evidence to suggest that they influence the outcome of recently induced complete heart block.

Ventricular dysrhythmias Ventricular extrasystoles are commonly a manifestation of potassium deficiency. If the results of analysis are not available immediately, a test dose of 5 mmol of potassium can be given, but doses in excess of 1 g KCl (13·6 mmol) should not be given unless there is biochemical evidence of depletion. Potassium replacement should be undertaken with particular care if the urinary output is low.

Ventricular excitability may persist when the plasma potassium concentration is normal. Lignocaine (1–2 mg/kg) as a bolus or an infusion of 1 mg/min may suppress the ectopic focus. Ventricular tachycardia during the closing stages of bypass often indicates severe myocardial damage, and even small doses of β-adrenergic blocking agents should be avoided because asystole can easily occur if myocardial function is depressed any further. The treatment of choice for ventricular tachycardia is DC defibrillation (25–100 J), followed if necessary by an infusion of lignocaine (1 mg/min).

Supraventricular dysrhythmias The cardiac output is sometimes critically dependent upon the presence of normal atrial systole, especially in patients with aortic valve disease. Atrial fibrillation, flutter, or nodal rhythm prevent satisfactory ventricular filling, particularly if the ventricular rate is fast. A synchronised transatrial DC shock (12·5–25 J) often restores sinus rhythm; if a synchronised defibrillator is not available, a random shock of the same magnitude can be given but may produce ventricular fibrillation which then requires defibrillation with a larger shock. Patients with atrial fibrillation preoperatively can also be defibrillated at the time of operation, if the fibrillation was of recent onset and complete haemodynamic correction has been achieved. This should not be attempted in patients with long-standing atrial fibrillation, a few of whom may, however, be suitable for an attempt at elective cardioversion (p. 71) in the late postoperative period.

It is important to control the ventricular rate even when sinus rhythm cannot be restored. Digitalis is the drug of choice, the dose depending on whether or not the patient was digitalised preoperatively and when therapy was discontinued. The effects of digitalis are long-lasting, and it is preferable if possible to discontinue bypass before the drug is injected so that the entire dose is given to the patient, and not diluted to an unknown degree in the extracorporeal circuit. Some effect on ventricular function and heart rate will be apparent within 30 minutes of an intravenous injection of digoxin.

Supraventricular tachycardia can sometimes be eliminated with verapamil (1·25–5·0 mg); very occasionally, small doses of selective β-adrenergic blocking agents (e.g. oxprenolol 0·25–1.0 mg) can be used safely if the supraventricular dysrhythmia persists but ventricular function is otherwise good. Isoprenaline is the agent of choice for increasing the ventricular rate when there is nodal bradycardia.

Termination of cardiopulmonary bypass

It should be possible to discontinue cardiopulmonary bypass as soon as the heart is beating in a stable rhythm at an acceptable rate. The caval snares are released and the venous cannulae are withdrawn into the right atrium and progressively obstructed so that a higher proportion of the systemic venous return enters the heart. At the same time the flow rate from the arterial pump is decreased. Pressure transients in time with the heart beat should then be superimposed on the perfusion pressure until ultimately an arterial pressure of normal configuration remains when the pump flow is stopped. If ventricular function is very poor, negligible or inadequate pressure transients appear, even though the heart is adequately filled (p. 97). The following measures should then be considered.

Myocardial support

In the first instance, bypass is continued while a biochemical survey is undertaken to exclude hypoxia, hypercapnia, metabolic acidosis or electrolyte abnormalities. While the results are awaited, mechanical causes of poor heart action (p. 91) are sought and corrected if possible. A relatively common cause is coronary air embolism which can profoundly impair myocardial function and cause persistent dysrhythmias. Sometimes air bubbles are visible in the coronary vessels and abrupt changes in the ECG occur at the same time. Fortunately, the effects of coronary air embolism are relatively short-lived and satisfactory ventricular function generally returns after 15 to 60 minutes of good coronary perfusion.

Prolonged perfusion of an undisturbed, non-distended heart as described on pp. 92 and 96 often allows non-specific myocardial damage to recover sufficiently for the ventricles to be able to support the circulation. Improvement is indicated if a previously abnormal, often ischaemic, ECG returns towards normal, and further evidence is obtained if the pressure in the left ventricular cavity is monitored through a needle inserted into the tubing of the left ventricular vent. Drainage through the vent prevents left ventricular distension and there is little or no ejection through the aortic valve, but pressure *is* developed within the chamber during each contraction. The magnitude and rate of rise of pressure, the effects of transitorily increasing the filling pressure (by momentarily occluding the venous drainage), or of giving inotropic drugs (see below), can all be monitored more readily than if progress is judged solely by the ECG, the appearance of the heart, and the magnitude of pressure transients on the arterial waveform.

Inotropic drugs are often invaluable at this stage. Adrenaline has both α and β stimulant properties whereas isoprenaline is a purely β-adrenergic agonist and is preferred in the first place. The response of the heart to a bolus dose of 2–3 μg of isoprenaline is assessed; if little or no improvement is seen,

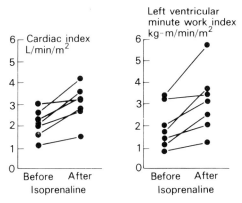

Figure 6.6 The effect of isoprenaline on ventricular function in a group of patients following open heart surgery. Reproduced from Jenkins *et al.*, 1973, by permission of the Editor, *Cardiovascular Research.*

the dose can be increased up to 10 or even 50 µg. The absence of a response to a dose of this magnitude implies that the ventricle is severely damaged and recovery may be impossible. Occasionally, doses of isoprenaline totalling several mg are used when β-adrenergic blockade persists from preoperative therapy.

The use of isoprenaline is sometimes limited by the development of an intolerable tachycardia whereas this occurs less frequently with adrenaline. Ventricular function may improve with adrenaline (10–100 µg) when iso-prenaline is ineffective, perhaps because it is both a powerful inotropic agent and also increases systemic vascular resistance, so raising the pressure at which the coronary arteries are perfused. Its chief disadvantage is that systemic vasoconstriction is inevitable.

Calcium chloride (1–5 mmol) is a myocardial stimulant which is effective whether or not the plasma concentration of ionised calcium is normal. A particularly powerful combination is adrenaline followed immediately by calcium chloride. The disadvantage of calcium salts is the risk of provoking ventricular dysrhythmias, especially if potassium equilibrium is disturbed.

Glucagon (0·5–1·0 mg initially) will sometimes improve myocardial performance, particularly if β-adrenergic blocking agents render isoprenaline or adrenaline ineffective. Part of the increase in cardiac output which follows its use has been attributed to peripheral circulatory effects, but it also has a direct action on the myocardium. The effect of a single injection lasts 30 to 40 minutes.

Large doses of corticosteroids (e.g. methyl prednisolone, 30 mg/kg) are sometimes given when myocardial function is failing. It is argued that they stabilise cell and lysosomal membranes, but evidence for their efficacy on the damaged myocardium is scanty.

The effects of some adrenergic agents (e.g. salbutamol, low doses of dopamine) are predominantly on the peripheral circulation. They are therefore of little value when the peripheral circulation is maintained by cardiopulmonary bypass, although a transition from isoprenaline or adrenaline may be indicated once bypass has been discontinued successfully.

Prolonged supportive perfusion, continued if necessary for several hours and supplemented with inotropic agents, may improve myocardial function to such an extent that the heart can once again support the circulation. The benefit of the technique is probably due to the passage of time after relief of the initial noxious stimulus, together with good coronary perfusion at a head of pressure sufficient to overcome the resistance of diseased arteries, and the elimination of ventricular work.

The concept of maintaining good diastolic perfusion through the coronary system while relieving the ventricle of excessive work has led to the development of aortic counter-pulsation or 'balloon pumping'. An inflatable balloon is inserted from one femoral artery high into the aorta. Carbon dioxide or helium is used to inflate the balloon during diastole at a frequency which is locked to the heart rate by using the R wave of the ECG to trigger the start of each cycle. The inflated balloon prevents blood leaving the ascending aorta, the diastolic fall in aortic blood pressure is arrested and a good flow at a high pressure is driven through the coronary arteries. The balloon is deflated during ventricular systole, so diminishing the afterload; ventricular work decreases and the stroke volume rises.

Aortic counter-pulsation has been advocated as a means of support for patients with severe myocardial failure following open heart surgery. The recovery rate of those who cannot sustain an effective circulation without mechanical aid is very low, but if counter-pulsation is to be used the optimum time for starting it is when the heart action is still barely sufficient to sustain an adequate circulation in spite of prolonged cardiopulmonary bypass and inotropic therapy.

MANAGEMENT IN THE IMMEDIATE POSTPERFUSION PERIOD

The majority of patients do not require the techniques described in the previous section. Once the heart is beating well the left ventricular vent is clamped and removed, and cardiotomy sites are inspected to confirm that there is no significant bleeding. It is easier to do this while bypass continues because distorting the heart to gain access to the posterior or posterolateral surfaces disturbs the ventricle and prevents it filling

Return of an optimum blood volume

Bypass is discontinued as described on p. 94, the volume of blood transferred to the patient being judged by the height of the venous pressures, the level of the arterial pressure, and the appearance of the heart.

The relationship between the force of contraction of a failing heart and the degree of cardiac filling has been discussed in detail in Chapter 1, where it was noted that until myocardial failure is severe, the force of contraction increases, at least to some extent, as the filling pressure is raised. Cardiac filling and hence cardiac output tend to fall in the immediate postperfusion period because blood loss continues, peripheral vasodilatation is occurring, particularly if rewarming has been incomplete during bypass, and the intravascular volume is contracting as the electrolyte load from the extracorporeal circuit is redistributed and excreted. For these reasons, it is desirable to keep the heart fairly full. When myocardial function is excellent, a normal cardiac output and arterial pressure are generated when the left and right atrial pressures are approximately 10 and 5 mm Hg (1·3 and 0·7 kPa) respectively, relative to the mid-axillary line. Overdistension causes unnecessarily vigorous cardiac contraction and systemic hypertension.

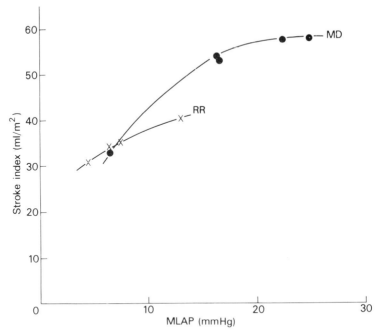

Figure 6.7 Left ventricular function following mitral valve replacement: male aged 30 (RR) compared with a normal (MD). The relationship between stroke index and mean left atrial pressure (MLAP) referred to zero at the *sternal angle* is shown.

When myocardial function is impaired, an acceptable cardiac output can only be generated if the atrial pressures are abnormally elevated. If the function of both ventricles is moderately impaired but to a comparable degree, it may be necessary to increase cardiac filling until the left atrial pressure is between 15 and 20 mm Hg (2·0 and 2·7 kPa) relative to the mid-axillary line and the right atrial pressure is a few mm lower. Any inequality of function on the two sides of the heart will be apparent as a discrepancy between the atrial pressures as discussed on p. 5, and if right ventricular failure predominates the right atrial pressure will be the higher of the two.

When heart failure is severe, it is customary to increase the higher of the two atrial pressures to between 20 and 25 mm Hg (2·7 and 3·3 kPa) relative to the mid-axillary line in the hope of obtaining maximum benefit from the heterometric response (p. 4). Higher pressures do not increase the stroke output and may cause it to fail if distension permits regurgitation across the atrioventricular valves (p. 112).

Elevation of the atrial pressures to this extent causes 'back pressure' effects as described on pp. 11 and 15, and it is important to note that oedema accumulates readily following bypass because the plasma protein concentration has been lowered by haemodilution and there is capillary damage, particularly in the lungs.

Reversal of heparin

The caval cannulae are removed as soon as it is apparent that a satisfactory circulation has been restored and that there is no major source of bleeding. The arterial cannula is not necessarily removed at the same time because it provides a route through which filtered, warm blood, albeit anticoagulated with heparin, can be given quickly should the need arise.

Protamine sulphate is given to reverse the effects of heparin after the venous cannulae have been removed. The continued presence of the arterial cannula is not a contraindication, but the suckers which return blood to the oxygenator can no longer be used because entry of blood containing protamine causes clot formation in the oxygenator. Unless tests of heparin activity are readily available, it is generally assumed that a constant degree of heparinisation has been maintained throughout perfusion and the dose of protamine is calculated as approximately twice that of the initial dose of heparin.

Protamine must always be injected slowly over a period of ten to fifteen minutes. It is a myocardial depressant and causes both peripheral vasodilatation and pulmonary vasoconstriction. Hypotension following the administration of protamine is caused most commonly by peripheral vasodilatation and is therefore likely to occur in patients who are relatively hypovolaemic but vasoconstricted because they are still slightly cold, or have been treated with adrenaline. Both the right and left atrial pressures drop at the same time as the blood pressure, and rapid transfusion rapidly restores cardiac filling and a satisfactory output. If necessary, blood can be returned from the extra-corporeal circuit through the arterial line.

The administration of protamine to patients with severe pulmonary vascular disease is much more hazardous. A further rise in the already elevated pulmonary vascular resistance may prevent the right ventricle ejecting effectively; the right atrial pressure rises while the left atrial pressure and hence the blood pressure fall rapidly. Isoprenaline is a pulmonary vasodilator as well as a myocardial stimulant and $2-10\,\mu g$ should be given immediately, even if an infusion of isoprenaline is already in progress. At the same time, 100% oxygen is given for a few minutes. If these measures fail to restore blood flow through the lungs, it may be necessary to re-establish cardiopulmonary bypass. Extra heparin is given and at least one venous cannula is quickly reintroduced into the distended right atrium. Bypass is continued until the right ventricle has recovered; the venous cannulae are removed once more and the required dose of protamine is given in minute doses (10–20 mg at a time) over a prolonged period.

PRESERVATION OF A STABLE CIRCULATION

Blood transfusion

Blood is transfused to maintain optimal atrial pressures as determined at the end of bypass (p. 97); for reasons noted already, the volume required is often in excess of the measured loss. Sometimes the venous pressures fall during the first few hours after bypass without detriment to the circulation. This indicates progressive improvement in myocardial function and is not an indication for rapid transfusion, provided there is no evidence of active blood loss, the arterial pressure is good, the urine output well maintained and the peripheral circulation dilated so that even the legs and feet feel warm to the touch.

The blood and electrolyte mixture in the oxygenator is sometimes returned slowly if no stored blood has been added during bypass because part of the patient's original blood volume has been transferred to the extra-corporeal apparatus. Unless this is returned, or replaced with an equal volume of stored blood, hypovolaemia will tend to occur as the aliquot of electrolyte solution in the patient is redistributed and excreted, and anaemia will become apparent in the postoperative period. Blood damage occurs during perfusion, and it may be wiser to discard the contents of the oxygenator and use stored blood if bypass was particularly prolonged or was accompanied by an unusual amount of intracardiac suction. If blood from the oxygenator *is* used, 50 mg of protamine should be given to neutralise the heparin in each 500 ml.

Hyperkalemia, metabolic acidosis and the infusion of platelet and white cell debris are all less likely to follow transfusion of the relatively fresh blood which is generally available for open heart surgery. A blood warmer should be used if rapid transfusion is required, and calcium salts may be needed if ACD or CPD blood is given quickly. It is desirable to incorporate small pore filters in the infusion line, particularly if massive transfusion is necessary or if there is pre-existing pulmonary pathology.

Drug therapy

Many patients require inotropic agents as well as considerable elevation of cardiac filling pressures. Isoprenaline and occasionally adrenaline are continued after bypass, preferably by infusion at a dose which is usually between 1 and 5 μg/minute. Isoprenaline induces peripheral vasodilatation, and both atrial pressures commonly fall when the infusion is started. The systolic blood pressure increases if the heart is capable of responding to inotropic stimulation, provided the simultaneous elevation of heart rate is not extreme. The diastolic blood pressure remains unchanged or may fall a little. Adrenaline

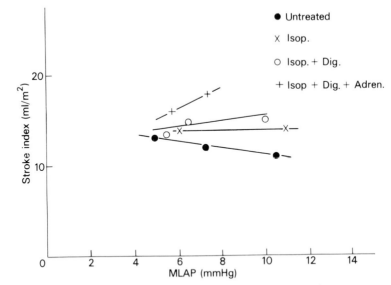

Figure 6.8   The effect of pharmacological support on a failing left ventricle following open heart surgery. The apparent downward slope of the ventricular function curve before treatment probably indicates a diminution in forward flow caused by atrio-ventricular valve regurgitation. The left atrial pressure (MLAP) was referred to zero at the *sternal angle*. Isop. = isoprenaline; Dig. = digoxin; Adren. = adrenaline.

is preferred if isoprenaline is ineffective or causes an unacceptable tachycardia; it can be regarded as the drug of first choice if a high diastolic blood pressure is considered essential, but it too can increase the heart rate and ventricular excitability. A reflex bradycardia secondary to hypertension is uncommon. Dobutamine, a fairly selective β-adrenergic stimulant with inotropic but little chronotropic activity may prove to be a valuable agent.

Salbutamol is sometimes selected in preference to isoprenaline. Although 1000 times less potent than isoprenaline as an inotropic agent, it is only 2–5 times less potent as a peripheral vasodilator. Relatively large doses can therefore be given to induce arteriolar dilatation without increasing the cardiac rate or excitability. Cardiac work and myocardial oxygen consumption remain unchanged but the cardiac output rises as the systemic vascular resistance falls. Unlike many drugs used to lower peripheral resistance, venodilatation is not a prominent feature and transfusion requirements do not increase. For this reason, it is much easier to use than the various α-adrenergic blocking agents or sodium nitroprusside which have been advocated to decrease the after-load on the left ventricle, and hence improve the cardiac output without augmenting contractility or increasing myocardial oxygen requirements.

Dopamine has achieved some recent popularity. At low doses ($2 \cdot 5 \, \mu g/kg/min$) the chief effect is a selective increase in renal and mesenteric blood flow. At higher rates of infusion ($5–10 \, \mu g/kg/min$) an inotropic effect can be demonstrated too, and above $15 \, \mu g/kg/min$ peripheral vasoconstriction is apparent.

These drugs are all given by infusion, and if large doses are required over prolonged periods excessive amounts of the diluent will be given too. The use of concentrated solutions avoids this hazard, but these must be controlled very carefully to prevent a sudden large bolus reaching the patient inadvertently. Isoprenaline and adrenaline are commonly diluted in 5% dextrose solution, 1 mg in 100 ml; an infusion rate of 8 drops per minute from a standard giving set provides approximately $5 \, \mu g$ of the drug per minute and 30 ml of dextrose solution per hour. Salbutamol (20 mg in 500 ml) is generally infused at a rate of $10–30 \, \mu g/minute$, and dopamine (200–400 mg in 500 ml) at a rate which varies according to the effect required. An infusion pump, automatic drip counter or microdrip apparatus increases the accuracy and safety of drug administration.

Continued potassium replacement is generally necessary, and potassium chloride should be given intravenously at a rate of 10 mmol of potassium for every 200 ml of urine passed. Concentrated potassium salts must also be given slowly, for example 1 g KCl (13·6 mmol K) over 15 minutes. Patients with a preoperative deficit may require larger quantities whereas those who have never been treated with diuretics and who have had a short bypass can be managed safely if potassium replacement is delayed until the operation has been completed and the remainder of the 24-hour fluid and electrolyte requirement is being prescribed.

A metabolic acidosis is sometimes detected in the postperfusion period, particularly after profound hypothermia and circulatory arrest, or if there has been a prolonged period of circulatory inadequacy. Lactic acid is metabolised readily by well-perfused, normothermic tissues, and the acidosis is often transitory once a satisfactory circulation has been restored. By comparison, bicarbonate is excreted relatively slowly and unnecessary doses of sodium bicarbonate should be avoided, particularly as the common finding after uncomplicated open heart surgery is a metabolic alkalosis caused by the metabolism of citrate in ACD or CPD blood. In addition, rapid infusion of sodium bicarbonate can provoke fatal dysrhythmias, possibly because tissue oxygenation is impaired by the alkali-induced shift in the oxygen–haemoglobin dissociation curve. A base deficit of 5 mmol/l or less in an otherwise well patient is probably best left alone.

Sodium bicarbonate should be given if a metabolic acidosis is present and the state of the circulation is unsatisfactory. It is sometimes difficult to select an appropriate dose because the degree of acidosis depends upon both the extent of perfusion of peripheral tissues and biochemical changes such as those described above which are going on simultaneously. The formula [dose of bicarbonate in mmol $= \frac{1}{3}$ (base deficit × body weight in kg)] often suggests an amount which proves to be excessive, and half this amount should be given in the first instance. Alternatively, the dose can be calculated empirically according to the formula [base deficit × presumptive blood volume (0·08 l/kg)]. Subsequent measurements will determine whether or not further doses are required but an overdose is unlikely if this regime is followed.

Ventilation

Pulmonary damage is a sequel of cardiopulmonary bypass (see Chapter 9). Gas exchange may also be impaired by the deleterious effects of massive blood transfusion or the pulmonary complications of cardiac failure. It is sometimes necessary to raise the inspired oxygen concentration to ensure an arterial oxygen tension in excess of 12 kPa; positive end-expiratory pressure may be helpful and is unlikely to influence cardiac output while the chest is open. The minute volume has to be increased occasionally to maintain a normal arterial carbon dioxide tension, but this is only common for the first 30 to 60 minutes after profound hypothermia while the carbon dioxide retained at low temperatures is excreted.

UNEXPECTED CARDIAC ARREST IN THE POSTPERFUSION PERIOD

Sudden changes of rhythm may occur spontaneously or may follow mechanical disturbance to the heart or coronary vessels while haemostasis is being secured. Sometimes there is a biochemical or pharmacological cause such as potassium salts given too rapidly or in excessive dosage, or the sudden infusion of a large bolus of adrenaline or isoprenaline. Cardiac massage and efficient oxygenation are required as usual, but sodium bicarbonate is not always necessary if the heart beat is restored quickly. If the chest has already been closed, the sternum should be reopened and internal massage continued in case there is some mechanical problem within the pericardial cavity. If the heart cannot be restarted rapidly, it may be necessary to re-establish cardiopulmonary bypass while the cause of the arrest is determined and treated. When bypass is required again after the administration of protamine has been completed, it is wise to use a twice normal dose of heparin to ensure that clotting does not occur within the extracorporeal apparatus. Subsequent management will depend on the cause of the arrest.

CLOSURE OF THE CHEST

Chest drains are positioned in front and behind the heart and pass through separate incisions in the chest wall to graduated cylinders in which continued blood loss can be collected and measured. Suction is applied as soon as the incision is air-tight, to prevent blood or clot accumulating inside the pericardial sac. Pleural drains are required too if these cavities have been opened.

Closure of the pericardium can restrict the movement of the heart if it is dilated or overfull; a transitory fall in arterial pressure occurs and the atrial pressures rise. These changes rarely persist, but may do so if cardiac function is very poor. The pericardial cavity can be left open if the heart has been approached through a median sternotomy, but dense adhesions are likely to develop and will impede access if cardiac surgery is ever required again.

Closing the sternum can sometimes produce similar changes in the atrial and arterial pressures. The arterial pressure generally recovers by the time the incision is closed, but the atrial pressures now reflect the positive intrathoracic pressure of controlled ventilation and will remain a little higher than when the chest was open.

TRANSFER TO THE INTENSIVE CARE UNIT

This is one of the more dangerous periods of open heart surgery. The patient is disconnected from the drainage cylinders and from some at least of the monitoring apparatus; physical movement and sometimes the return of consciousness are both disturbing features while new staff are commonly responsible for subsequent management.

The drains should be disconnected for the minimum possible time, and haemodynamic monitoring is retained until the patient is ready to be moved from the operating table to the bed. Pacemaker wires and monitoring lines emerging through the chest wall are strapped to the chest and suitably labelled. The availability of battery-operated ECG monitors ensures that cardiac rhythm and rate at least can be followed without interruption.

IPPV is virtually always required postoperatively. Muscle relaxants are therefore not reversed at the end of the operation and the patient is sedated to ensure there is no coughing or straining during transfer.

Gastric secretions accumulate during operation, particularly in patients with a high systemic venous pressure. A nasogastric tube should be passed while the patient is still unconscious to prevent discomfort and retching during the period of postoperative IPPV.

A portable oxygen cylinder carried on the bed can be used to permit manual ventilation during the journey. Alternatively, the anaesthetic machine can be wheeled behind the bed, but this is only feasible if the Intensive Care Unit is close to the theatre.

If the patient is not accompanied by a member of the operating theatre team, it is essential for a full account of the current position to be given at the time of transfer, together with written instructions for subsequent management.

PRINCIPLES OF POSTOPERATIVE CARE

The details of postoperative management are not discussed in this text but the principles are based upon a continuation of the care provided in the postperfusion period. They can be listed as:

1 Maintenance of optimum blood volume (pp. 97 and 99).
2 Provision of pharmacological or, occasionally, mechanical support for the circulation, aiming to achieve a satisfactory perfusion pressure as well as an appropriate distribution of blood flow to individual organs (pp. 94 and 100).
3 Control of dysrhythmias (p. 92).
4 Attention to fluid and electrolyte requirements and acid-base balance,

bearing in mind the need to promote the excretion of crystalloid solutions used during perfusion and the tendency to hyperglycaemia (p. 22), hypo-kalaemia (p. 83) and metabolic alkalosis (p. 102).

5 Continuation of controlled ventilation until the circulation is stable and satisfactory, the body temperature is normal and arterial blood gas tensions within the normal range can be achieved easily with only moderate oxygen-enrichment of the inspired air (e.g. not more than 40%).

The resumption of spontaneous ventilation and extubation can follow surgery in many patients within a few hours of their return to the Intensive Care Unit. If in doubt about the ability of a patient to sustain the effort of breathing spontaneously, a short trial with the endotracheal tube in place is often helpful. Unfavourable signs in the spontaneously breathing patient are any elevation of either atrial pressure, an increase in heart rate or the appearance of a dysrhythmia, reduction in the urine output, tachypnoea, sweating or restlessness, and any change in blood pressure other than an abrupt increase with the cessation of intermittent positive pressure ventilation. Measurements of arterial blood gas tensions are rarely helpful, and the decision to re-establish controlled ventilation is usually taken on clinical grounds. If attempts at spontaneous ventilation are unsuccessful, further measures will be required to improve either cardiac or respiratory function. Measures to be considered which are of particular relevance to pulmonary function include the improvement of pleural drainage, re-expansion of atelectatic areas, the use of bronchodilator drugs if necessary, and the application of positive end-expiratory pressure if it is difficult to maintain a satisfactory arterial oxygen tension because of generalised pulmonary (alveolar) pathology. Some patients can be weaned most easily from IPPV to spontaneous ventilation via a period of spontaneous ventilation with continuous positive airway pressure.

The postoperative course is not always straightforward and the complications of open heart surgery are discussed in Chapter 10.

REFERENCES

The references relating to the following topics are listed in Chapter 5:

General principles of anaesthesia for cardiac surgery

Muscle relaxants and their reversal

Effects of controlled ventilation

Humidification of the respiratory tract

EFFECTS OF GENERAL ANAESTHETIC AGENTS AND TECHNIQUES

BERTOLO A., NOVAKOVIC L. & PENNA M. (1972) Anti-arrhythmic effects of droperidol. *Anesthesiology* **37**, 529

BROADLEY J. N. & TAYLOR P. A. (1974) An assessment of Althesin for the induction of anaesthesia in cardiac surgical patients: a comparison with thiopentone. *British Journal of Anaesthesia* **46**, 687.

BROWN B. R. Jr. & CROUT J. R. (1971) A comparative study of the effects of five general anesthetics on myocardial contractility. *Anesthesiology* **34**, 236.

CONAHAN T. J., OMINSKY A. J., WOLLMAN H. & STROTH R. A. (1973) A prospective random comparison of halothane and morphine for open heart anesthesia. *Anesthesiology* **38**, 528.

CÔTÉ P., GUÉRET P. & BOURASSA M. G. (1974) Systemic and coronary hemodynamic effects of diazepam with normal and diseased coronary arteries. *Circulation* **50**, 1210.

HARRISON S. G. C. & SELLICK B. A. (1972) Cardiovascular effects of Althesin in patients with cardiac pathology: a preliminary communication. *British Journal of Anaesthesia* **44**, 1205.

LAPPAS D. G., BUCKLEY M. J., LAVER M. B., DAGGETT W. M. & LOWENSTEIN E. (1975) Left ventricular performance and pulmonary circulation following addition of nitrous oxide to morphine during coronary artery surgery. *Anesthesiology* **43**, 61.

LAPPAS D. G., GEHA D., FISHER J. E., LAVER M. B. & LOWENSTEIN E. (1975) Filling pressures of the heart and pulmonary circulation of the patient with coronary artery disease after large intravenous doses of morphine. *Anesthesiology* **42**, 153.

LILLEASSEN P., AUNE J. & STOVNER J. (1975) Ketamine-pancuronium induction in patients with aortic stenosis. *Acta Anaesthesiologica Scandinavica* **19**, 193.

LOWENSTEIN E., HALLOWELL P., LEVINE F. M., DAGGETT W. M., AUSTEN W. G. & LAVER M. B. (1969) Cardiovascular response to large doses of intravenous morphine in man. *New England Journal of Medicine* **281**, 1389.

LOWENSTEIN E. (1971) Morphine 'anesthesia': a perspective. *Anesthesiology* **35**, 565.

LYONS S. M. & CLARKE R. S. J. (1972) A comparison of different drugs for anaesthesia in cardiac surgical patients. *British Journal of Anaesthesia* **44**, 575.

McDERMOTT R. W. & STANLEY T. H. (1974) The cardiovascular effects of low concentrations of nitrous oxide during morphine anesthesia. *Anesthesiology* **41**, 89.

MOFFITT E. A., TARHAN S., RODRIGUEZ R., BARNHORST D. A. & PLUTH J. R. (1976) Hemodynamic effects of morphine during and early after cardiac operations. *Current Researches in Anesthesia and Analgesia* **55**, 47.

MORGAN M., LUMLEY J. & GILLIES I. D. S. (1974) Neuroleptanaesthesia for major surgery: experience with 500 cases. *British Journal of Anaesthesia* **46**, 288.

NGAI S. H., MARK L. C. & PAPPER E. M. (1970) Pharmacologic and physiologic aspects of anesthesiology. *New England Journal of Medicine* **282**, 479 & 541.

PRICE H. L. (1976) Myocardial depression by nitrous oxide and its reversal by Ca^{++}. *Anesthesiology* **44**, 211.

PRICE H. L., COOPERMAN L. H., WARDEN J. C., MORRIS J. J. & SMITH T. C. (1969) Pulmonary hemodynamics during general anesthesia in man. *Anesthesiology* **30**, 629.

SHIMOSATO S., YASUDA I., KEMMOTSU O., SHANKS C. & GAMBLE C. (1973) Effect of halothane on altered contractility of isolated heart muscle obtained from cats with experimentally produced ventricular hypertrophy and failure. British *Journal of Anaesthesia* **45**, 2.

STANLEY T. H., BENNETT G. M., LOESER E. A., KAWAMURA R. & SENTKER C. R. (1976) Cardiovascular effects of diazepam and droperidol during morphine anesthesia. *Anesthesiology* **44**, 255.

STOELTING R. K. & GIBBS P. S. (1973) Hemodynamic effects of morphine and morphine-nitrous oxide in valvular heart disease and coronary artery disease. *Anesthesiology* **38**, 45.

STOELTING R. K., GIBBS P. S., CREASSER C. W. & PETERSON C. (1975) Hemodynamic and ventilatory responses to fentanyl, fentanyl-droperidol, and nitrous oxide in patients with acquired valvular heart disease. *Anesthesiology* **42**, 319.

STOELTING R. K., REIS R. R. & LONGNECKER D. E. (1972) Hemodynamic responses to nitrous oxide-halothane and halothane in patients with valvular heart disease. *Anesthesiology* **37**, 430.

THORNTON J. A., FLEMING J. S., GOLDBERG A. D. & BAIRD D. (1973) Cardiovascular effects of 50% nitrous oxide and 50% oxygen mixture. *Anaesthesia* **28**, 484.

WHITWAM J. G. & RUSSELL W. J. (1971) The acute cardiovascular changes and adrenergic blockade by droperidol in man. *British Journal of Anaesthesia* **43**, 581.

WONG K. C., MARTIN W. E., HORNBEIN T. F., FREUND F. G. & EVERETT J. (1973) The cardiovascular effects of morphine sulfate with oxygen and with nitrous oxide in man. *Anesthesiology* **38**, 542.

MONITORING

Arterial cannulation

ALLEN E. V. (1929) Thromboangiitis obliterans: methods of diagnosis of chronic occlusive arterial lesions distal to the wrist, with illustrative cases, *American Journal of Medical Science* **178**, 237.

BARBER J. D., WRIGHT D. J. & ELLIS R. H. (1973) Radial artery puncture: a simple screening test of the ulnar anastomotic circulation. *Anaesthesia* **28**, 291.

BEDFORD R. F. & WOLLMAN H. (1973) Complications of percutaneous radial artery cannulation: an objective, prospective study in man. *Anesthesiology* **38**, 228.

BEDFORD R. F. (1975) Percutaneous radial artery cannulation—increased safety using Teflon catheters. *Anesthesiology* **42**, 219.

DOWNES J. B., RACKSTEIN A. D., KLEIN E. F. Jr. & HAWKINS I. F. Jr. (1973) Hazards of radial artery catheterization. *Anesthesiology* **38**, 283.

KIM J. M., ARAKAWA K. & BLISS J. (1975) Arterial cannulation: factors in the development of occlusion. *Current Researches in Anesthesia and Analgesia* **54**, 836.

RAMANATHAN S., CHALON J. & TURNDORF J. (1975) Determining patency of palmar arches by retrograde radial pulsation. *Anesthesiology* **42**, 756.

Central venous pressure and oxygenation of mixed venous blood

ARMSTRONG R. F., SOUTHORN P. A., SECKER-WALKER J., LINCOLN J. C. R. & SOUTTER L. (1976) Continuous monitoring of mixed venous oxygen tension. *British Medical Journal* **3**, 282.

BRISCOE C. E. (1973) A comparison of jugular and central venous pressure measurements during anaesthesia. *British Journal of Anaesthesia* **45**, 173.

DAVIDSON J. T., BEN HUR N. & NATHEN H. (1963) Subclavian venipuncture. *Lancet* **2**, 1139.

ENGLISH I. C. W., FREW R. M., PIGGOTT J. F. & ZAKI M. (1969) Percutaneous catheterisation of the internal jugular vein. *Anaesthesia* **24**, 521.

KRAUSS X. H., VERDOUW P. D., HUGENHOLTZ P. G. & NAUTA J. (1975) On-line monitoring of mixed venous oxygen saturation after cardiothoracic surgery. *Thorax* **30**, 636.

LEE J., WRIGHT F., BARBER R. & STANLEY L. (1972) Central venous oxygen saturation in shock: a study in man. *Anesthesiology* **36**, 472.

SCHEINMAN M. M., BROWN M. A. & RAPAPORT E. (1969) Critical assessment of use of central venous oxygen saturation as a mirror of mixed venous oxygen in severely ill cardiac patients. *Circulation* **40**, 165.

STOELTING R. K. (1973) Evaluation of external jugular venous pressure as a reflection of right atrial pressure. *Anesthesiology* **38**, 291.

YOFFA D. (1965) Supraclavicular subclavian venipuncture and catheterization. *Lancet* **2**, 614.

Temperature

WHITBY J. D. & DUNKIN L. J. (1971) Cerebral, oesophageal and nasopharyngeal temperatures. *British Journal of Anaesthesia* **43**, 673.

Cerebral electrical activity

BRANTHWAITE M. A. (1973) Detection of neurological damage during open heart surgery. *Thorax* **28**, 464.
BRANTHWAITE M. A. (1973) Factors affecting cerebral activity during open heart surgery. *Anaesthesia* **28**, 619.
JUNEJA I., FLYNN R. E. & BERGER R. L. (1972) The arterial and venous pressures, and the electroencephalogram during open heart surgery. *Acta Neurologica Scandinavica* **48**, 163.
SCHWARTZ M. S., COLVIN M. P., PRIOR P. F., STRUNLIN L., SIMPSON B. R., WEAVER E. J. M. & SCOTT D. F. (1973) The cerebral function monitor: its value in predicting the neurological outcome in patients undergoing cardiopulmonary bypass. *Anaesthesia* **28**, 611.

CONTROL OF COAGULATION

ELLISON N., OMINSKY A. J. & WOLLMAN H. (1971) Is protamine a clinically important anticoagulant? A negative answer. *Anesthesiology* **35**, 621.
FADALI M.A., PAPACOSTAS C.A., DUKE J. J., LEDBETTER M. & OSBAKKEN M. (1976) Cardiovascular depressant effect of protamine sulphate: experimental study and clinical implications. *Thorax* **31**, 320.
GUFFIN A. V., DUNBAR R. W., KAPLAN J. A. & BLAND J. W. Jr. (1976) Successful use of a reduced dose of protamine after cardiopulmonary bypass. *Current Researches in Anesthesia and Analgesia* **55**, 110.
JABERI M., BELL, W. R. & BENSON D. W. (1974) Control of heparin therapy in open heart surgery. *Journal of Thoracic and Cardiovascular Surgery* **67**, 133.
JASTRZEBSKI J., SYKES M. K. & WOODS D. G. (1974) Cardiorespiratory effects of protamine after cardiopulmonary bypass. *Thorax* **29**, 534.
RENO W. J., ROTMAN M., GRUMBINE F. C., DENNIS L. H. & MOHLER E. R. (1974) Control of heparin therapy in open heart surgery. *Journal of Thoracic and Cardiovascular Surgery* **67**, 133.
SCHRIEVER H. G., EPSTEIN S. E. & MINTZ M. D. (1973) Statistical correlation and heparin sensitivity of activated partial thromboplastin time, whole blood coagulation time, and an automated coagulation time. *American Journal of Clinical Pathology* **60**, 323.

CIRCULATORY SUPPORT AND THE CONTROL OF DYSRHYTHMIAS

Mechanical methods

BERGER R. L., SAINI V. K., RYAN T. J., SOKOL D. M. & KEEFE J. F. (1973) Intra-aortic balloon assist for postcardiotomy cardiogenic shock. *Journal of Thoracic and Cardiovascular Surgery* **66**, 906.
BRAIMBRIDGE M. V., CLEMENT A. J., YALAV E. & ERSOZ A. (1971) External DC defibrillation during open heart surgery. *Thorax* **26**, 455.
WISHEART J. D., WRIGHT J. E. C., ROSENFELDT F. L. & ROSS J. K. (1973) Atrial and ventricular pacing after open heart surgery. *Thorax* **28**, 9.

Pharmacological means

BEREGOVICH J., BIANCHI C., RUBLER S., LOMNITZ E., CAGIN N. & LEVITT B. (1974) Dose related hemodynamic and renal effects of dopamine in congestive heart failure. *American Heart Journal* **87**, 550.

BEREGOVICH J., REICHER-REISS H., KUNSTADT D. & GRISHMAN A. (1971) Hemodynamic effects of isoproterenol in cardiac surgery. *Journal of Thoracic and Cardiovascular Surgery* **62**, 957.

BROWN D. R. & STAREK P. (1974) Sodium nitroprusside induced improvement in cardiac function in association with left ventricular dilatation. *Anesthesiology* **41**, 521.

DALUZ P. L., FORRESTER J. S., WYATT H. L., TYBERG J. V., CHAGRASULIS R., PARMLEY W. W. & SWAN H. J. C. (1975). Hemodynamic and metabolic effects of sodium nitroprusside on the performance and metabolism of regional ischemic myocardium. *Circulation* **52**, 400.

EURENIUS S. & SMITH R. A. (1973) The effect of warming on the serum potassium content of stored blood. *Anesthesiology* **38**, 482.

FRANCIOSA J. A., GUIHA N. H., LIMAS C. J., RODRIGUERA E. & COHN J. N. (1972) Improved left ventricular function during nitroprusside infusion in acute myocardial infarction. *Lancet* **1**, 650.

GIBSON D. G. & COLTART D. J. (1971) Haemodynamic effects of intravenous salbutamol in patients with mitral valve disease: comparison with isoprenaline and atropine. *Postgraduate Medical Journal*, Supplement 47, 40.

GOLDBERG L. I. (1974) Dopamine: clinical use of an endogenous catecholamine. *New England Journal of Medicine* **291**, 707.

HAMER J., GIBSON D. & COLTART J. (1973) Effect of glucagon on left ventricular performance in aortic stenosis. *British Heart Journal* **35**, 312.

HOLLOWAY E. L., STINSON E. B., DERBY G. C. & HARRISON D. C. (1975) Action of drugs in patients early after cardiac surgery I: comparison of isoproterenol and dopamine. *American Journal of Cardiology* **35**, 656.

JENKINS B. S., BRANTHWAITE M. A. & BRADLEY R. D. (1973) Cardiac function after open heart surgery. *Cardiovascular Research* **7**, 297.

JEWITT D. E. (1975) Anti-arrhythmic drugs and their mechanisms of action. In *Modern Trends in Cardiology* **3**, Ed. M. F. Oliver, p. 333. Butterworth, London.

JEWITT D., BIRKHEAD J., MITCHELL A. & DOLLERY C. (1974). Clinical cardiovascular pharmacology of dobutamine, a selective inotropic catecholamine. *Lancet* **2**, 363.

Leading Article (1974) Sodium bicarbonate in cardiac arrest. *Lancet* **1**, 946.

LEIGHTON K. M. & BRUCE C. (1976) Dobutamine and general anaesthesia: a study of the response of arterial pressure, heart rate and renal blood flow. *Canadian Anaesthetists' Society Journal* **23**, 176.

MARINO R. J., TOMAGNOLI A. & KEATS A. S. (1975) Selective venoconstriction by dopamine in comparison with isoproterenol and phenylephrine. *Anesthesiology* **43**, 570.

MENTZNER R. M. Jr., ALEGRE C. A. & NOLAN S. P. (1976) The effects of dopamine and isoproterenol on the pulmonary circulation. *Journal of Thoracic and Cardiovascular Surgery* **71**, 807.

MURTAGH J. G., BINNION P. F., LAL S., HUTCHISON K. J. & FLETCHER E. (1970) Haemodynamic effects of glucagon. *British Heart Journal* **32**, 307.

REUL G. J. Jr., ROMAGNOLI A., SANDIFORD F. M., WUKASCH D. C., COOLEY D. A. & NORMAN J. C. (1974) Protective effect of propranolol on the hypertrophied heart during cardiopulmonary bypass. *Journal of Thoracic and Cardiovascular Surgery* **68**, 283.

SCHAMROTH L., KRIKLER D. M. & GARRETT C. (1972) Immediate effects of intravenous verapamil in cardiac arrhythmias. *British Medical Journal* **1**, 660.

SMITH G. H. & CHANDRA K. (1972) Haemodynamic effects of glucagon after mitral valve replacement. *Thorax* **27**, 591.

STAPENHORST K. (1970) The effect of some vasoactive drugs on the pulmonary circulation. *Abstract in Anesthesiology* **33,** 475. (Original reference: *Z. Ges. Exp. Med.* 1969, **151,** 103.)

TANAKA K. & PETTINGER W. A. (1973) Pharmokinetics of bolus potassium injections for cardiac arrhythmias. *Anesthesiology* **38,** 587.

TINKER J. H., TARHAN S., WHITE R. D., PLUTH J. R. & BARNHORST D. A. (1976) Dobutamine for inotropic support during emergence from cardiopulmonary bypass. *Anesthesiology* **44,** 281.

TY SMITH N. & CORBASCIO A. N. (1970) The use and misuse of pressor agents. *Anesthesiology* **33,** 58.

VANDER-ARK C. R. & REYNOLDS E. W. (1970) Effectiveness of glucagon in presence of beta-blockade. *American Heart Journal* **79,** 481.

WHITE R. D., GOLDSMITH R. S., RODRIGUEZ R., MOFFITT E. A. & PLUTH J. R. (1976) Plasma ionic calcium levels following injection of chloride, gluconate, and gluceptate salts of calcium. *Journal of Thoracic and Cardiovascular Surgery* **71,** 609.

WYSE S. D., GIBSON D. G. & BRANTHWAITE M. A. (1974) Haemodynamic effects of salbutamol in patients needing circulatory support after open heart surgery. *British Medical Journal* **3,** 502.

CHAPTER 7

IMPLICATIONS OF SOME SPECIFIC CONDITIONS

Chronic valve disease
Mitral valve disease
Aortic valve disease
Multiple valve replacement
Reoperation for valve disease
Ischaemic heart disease
Myocardial revascularisation
Resection of left ventricular aneurysm
Congenital heart disease
Closure of secundum atrial septal defect

Closure of ostium primum atrial septal defect
Closure of ventricular septal defect
Relief of pulmonary stenosis
Total correction of the tetralogy of Fallot
Glenn procedure for the relief of tricuspid atresia
Emergency open heart surgery
Pulmonary embolectomy

The principles which govern the management of patients during open heart surgery have been discussed in Chapter 6. Specific features which apply to individual conditions are described in this chapter with the intention of amplifying important aspects, rather than attempting to provide a comprehensive account. For this reason, the chapter can only be read intelligently as a sequel to Chapter 6.

CHRONIC VALVE DISEASE

Mitral valve disease

Mitral stenosis and/or incompetence usually follow rheumatic fever or chorea. Occasional patients present with mitral valve disease as an isolated congenital anomaly, and an increasing number are seen in middle age or later with mitral incompetence of relatively recent onset which is caused by papillary muscle dysfunction. Patients in this last category develop symptoms of pulmonary oedema early; sinus rhythm is often preserved and an exceptionally high 'v' wave in the left atrial pressure is characteristic (Fig. 7.1).

Those with rheumatic mitral valve disease develop symptoms more slowly, particularly if the valve is stenosed rather than incompetent. Gradual deterioration occurs over a number of years, often punctuated by episodes of increased disability related to the onset of atrial fibrillation, systemic embolism, or repeated infection of the respiratory tract. Restenosis after previous valvotomy is common, and calcification of the valve, myocardial fibrosis and obliterative pulmonary vascular disease are often present in older patients. Right ventricular failure, functional tricuspid incompetence and the consequences of systemic venous congestion mark the end stage of chronic mitral valve disease.

Patients with uncomplicated mitral stenosis can be relieved by closed valvotomy (p. 57) but those with significant incompetence, or with calcification of the valve require open heart surgery. Valve replacement is usually necessary although an incompetent valve can sometimes be repaired.

Many of these patients are seriously disabled, but they often tolerate the preliminary stages of anaesthesia and cardiac surgery surprisingly well. Premedication should be prescribed with caution for those with pulmonary disease complicating chronic pulmonary venous congestion, and drug dosage may need to be reduced for patients with systemic venous congestion or cardiac cachexia.

The right atrium is enormously distended in patients with long-standing right ventricular failure, and the venous pressures are very high. Moderate haemorrhage may occur while the chest is being opened, or during dissection

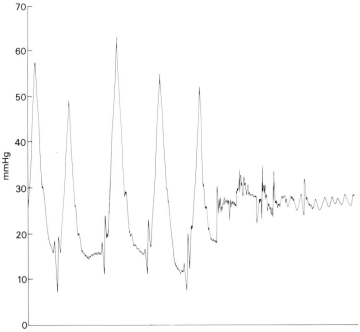

Figure 7.1 Dynamic and mean left atrial pressures in a male aged 67 with mitral incompetence caused by chordal rupture. In spite of the very high systolic peak pressure in the left atrium, the mean pressure was not high enough to generate significant pulmonary oedema and gas exchange was unimpaired.
Pressures are referred to zero at the mid-axillary line.

of the heart when there are dense adhesions following rheumatic pericarditis or previous surgery. Unless the haemorrhage is severe, blood loss before by-pass need not necessarily be replaced because the cardiac output is relatively independent of right atrial pressure and further distension of the right atrium merely increases the difficulty of cannulating the heart.

A common problem in the postperfusion period is the reappearance of tricuspid incompetence. This may have been present preoperatively but has often been abolished by bed rest and treatment with diuretics. It recurs if the heart is overdistended at the end of bypass or if myocardial function has been depressed, for example by prolonged ischaemia. Sometimes it resolves spontaneously, particularly if the atrial pressures can be allowed to fall a little; alternatively a small dose of isoprenaline (1–3 μg) can be given to improve myocardial tone. If these measures are ineffective, it may be necessary to pli-cate the tricuspid ring (tricuspid annuloplasty) or even replace the valve.

Intractable circulatory failure can occur in patients with severe pul-monary hypertension if the pulmonary vascular resistance increases any further during operation. Great care should be taken to avoid hypoxaemia, and protamine should be given with particular caution (p. 99). Pulmonary function is often disordered in those with chronic mitral valve disease and prolonged periods of artificial ventilation are often required in the postopera-tive period.

Aortic valve disease

Syncope, anginal pain and left ventricular failure are relatively early symptoms of aortic valve disease. Subsequent deterioration occurs fairly rapidly, and these patients usually present for treatment before permanent changes have occurred in the pulmonary vasculature. Severe congenital aortic stenosis is a cause of left ventricular failure in infancy (p. 178), while those with calcific

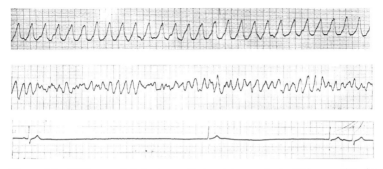

Figure 7.2 ECG recorded during a Stokes-Adams attack. This complex dys-rhythmia reverted spontaneously to sinus rhythm and the patient regained con-sciousness without treatment.

aortic stenosis are often in the older age groups and may have arterial disease elsewhere. They are therefore ill-equipped to withstand hypotension. Sometimes coronary arterial disease is present too, and coronary vein bypass grafting may be needed as well as aortic valve replacement.

An important distinction between patients with aortic valve disease and those with chronic mitral valve disease is that the former rarely develop atrial fibrillation. Indeed, the presence of this dysrhythmia in patients with aortic valve disease suggests that the mitral valve may be abnormal too and that the aetiology is probably rheumatic. Ventricular dysrhythmias or some form of heart block are more likely to be associated with pure aortic valve disease; Stokes-Adams attacks may occur and are sometimes transitory episodes of tachy-dysrhythmia rather than asystole or extreme bradycardia (Fig. 7.2).

Left ventricular function is good in a proportion of patients with aortic stenosis who require valve replacement as an elective, as distinct from an emergency procedure. When this is so, the left atrial and left ventricular end-diastolic pressures are within the normal range, and ventricular performance varies with end-diastolic fibre length in the normal way. The left ventricular stroke work is increased because a high intraventricular systolic pressure is required to maintain blood flow through the stenosed aortic valve, and the cardiac output may fall considerably if the diastolic stretch of the ventricular fibres is inadequate. These patients are therefore sensitive to quite small changes in blood volume; they are also critically dependent upon the preservation of sinus rhythm so that atrial systole can 'boost' ventricular filling and ensure adequate distension of the ventricle.

If aortic stenosis remains unrelieved, the cardiac output falls, the left ventricular end-diastolic pressure rises and pulmonary oedema may occur. Surgery can be required as a matter of urgency, and it is in this group that great care must be taken to avoid systemic vasodilatation. If the blood pressure falls when the cardiac output is fixed, coronary flow to the hypertrophied left ventricle is inadequate and asystole may occur. Minimal premedication, preoxygenation and induction with a minute dose of thiopentone or with intravenous diazepam are usually satisfactory.

Dilatation of the left ventricle and left ventricular failure occur relatively early in aortic regurgitation. The left ventricular stroke work is increased but it is the stroke volume rather than the pressure gradient which is high. Pulmonary oedema is often more prominent than diminished forward flow, and induction of anaesthesia is usually less hazardous than in patients with severe aortic stenosis. There is often a gross discrepancy between the atrial pressures on the two sides of the heart and transfusion should be undertaken cautiously, preferably with left atrial pressure monitoring established early in the course of operation so that hypotension caused by hypovolaemia can be distinguished from that due to worsening left ventricular failure. Knowledge of the left atrial pressure is also invaluable at the onset of perfusion when the degree of aortic regurgitation may be so great that a satisfactory mean arterial pressure cannot be maintained, and the left ventricle is unable to eject the volume of blood which enters its cavity. The ventricle distends, the left atrial pressure rises, and pulmonary damage will occur unless the distension is relieved by clamping the aorta and venting the left side of the heart.

Some patients have excellent myocardial function following aortic valve replacement, and hypertension can complicate the immediate postperfusion period, especially if the heart is overfull. This can be dangerous because the combination of a high blood pressure and a forcefully contracting left ventricle may disrupt the aortic suture line. Hypertension is less likely to occur if vasodilatation can be ensured and if the atrial pressures are raised no higher than is necessary to generate a satisfactory output at the end of perfusion (p. 97). If the blood pressure does rise too far, it can be lowered with intravenous phentolamine (1 mg initially); larger doses may have a profound hypotensive effect if the patient is vasoconstricted and therefore suffering from relative hypovolaemia.

Multiple valve replacement

Rheumatic heart disease often affects more than one valve. Mitral and aortic disease is a common combination, and mitral disease with either organic or functional impairment of the tricuspid valve is also common. Occasional patients require triple valve surgery but there is always reluctance to replace, as distinct from repair, the tricuspid valve because most tricuspid prostheses compromise right ventricular function to some extent.

It is sometimes impossible to determine preoperatively the extent to which individual valve lesions are responsible for disability. It may be necessary to replace or repair one valve and then restore the action of the heart before finally deciding whether or not to correct other valve lesions.

Numerous types of valve prosthesis are available, but the choice makes little difference to the conduct of anaesthesia. Thrombosis is less likely to

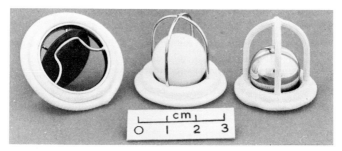

Figure 7.3 A selection of prosthetic valves. From left to right, these are a Björk-Shiley valve, a Starr-Edwards ball valve with silastic ball and metal cage, and a Starr-Edwards valve with metal ball and cloth-covered cage.

occur on tissue valves (homograft or heterograft) but is common on valves made of synthetic substances unless effective anticoagulation is instituted in the early postoperative period.

Reoperation for valve disease

Progression of the disease may necessitate reoperation in patients who have previously required closed or open cardiac surgery. Prosthetic valves may need to be replaced because of thrombosis, infection or separation of the prosthesis from the valve ring, or because degeneration of the substance of a biological (tissue) valve has rendered it incompetent.

The hazards of surgery are increased because haemorrhage is likely to occur from adhesions which follow previous operation, tissue planes cannot be identified easily and it is often difficult to mobilise the left ventricle sufficiently to insert the vent or evacuate air from its cavity. Reoperation is sometimes necessary as a mattery of urgency and special features of emergency surgery are considered on p. 125.

ISCHAEMIC HEART DISEASE

Myocardial revascularisation

The insertion of one or more aortocoronary arterial grafts, using a segment of the patient's own long saphenous vein, is now the technique of choice for the relief of anginal pain caused by localised obstruction within the coronary arterial system. Implantation of the internal mammary artery into the myocardium (Vineberg procedure) is virtually never performed at the present time.

Previous myocardial infarction is not a contraindication to surgery, indeed, revascularisation is sometimes undertaken immediately after infarction. The results of surgery in this group are no better than those of conservative management, and coronary vein bypass grafting tends to be reserved in the UK for patients who have angiographic evidence of localised obstruction in one or more coronary arteries and who suffer from disabling angina which persists in spite of medical treatment. Crescendo angina which may herald an episode of myocardial infarction is also an indication for surgery as soon as possible, provided there is an obstruction which can be bypassed.

Characteristically, patients with coronary arterial disease are much more anxious than those facing other forms of cardiac surgery. They may arrive in the anaesthetic room suffering from anginal pain unless heavy premedication has been prescribed. Prophylactic glyceryl trinitrate is sometimes given before transfer to the operating theatre, but ideally sedation should be sufficient to abolish anxiety. If anginal pain does occur, it can usually be relieved by the inhalation of 100% oxygen followed by additional sedation or the induction of anaesthesia.

Many of these patients have good left ventricular function and are quite robust. Doses of anaesthetic agents may need to be larger than those given to patients of comparable weight suffering from chronic valve disease. Sometimes, however, arterial disease is so severe that left ventricular function is uniformly poor, or there is a localised area of dyskinesia which prevents coordinated contraction. Impaired left ventricular function may not be apparent clinically if exercise tolerance is limited by pain before dyspnoea occurs. The performance of the ventricle is assessed radiologically during coronary arteriography and it is wise to note the findings before anaesthesia is induced.

Marked lability of the arterial blood pressure is another characteristic feature of patients with coronary arterial disease. Hypertension is common at the beginning of operation but can generally be controlled by deepening anaesthesia with halothane, narcotic analgesics or with droperidol. Intravenous glyceryl trinitrate (0·2–0·4 mg) is sometimes given to lower the blood-pressure and to promote coronary arterial vasodilatation. Attempts to lower the pressure must be undertaken cautiously because coronary perfusion can be inadequate if the diastolic pressure falls below a minimum critical value, and many of these patients also have arterial disease in other vascular beds. Changes in the ST segment of the ECG may provide early warning of a critically lowered diastolic pressure, and occur in some patients when the diastolic pressure is quite high (e.g. 75–80 mm Hg; 10–10·6 kPa). If the pressure falls below this level, coronary blood flow is decreased to such an extent that the heart may fail. Inotropic agents which do not increase the diastolic pressure (e.g. isoprenaline) are ineffective, and this is one of the few circumstances in which vasopressors are useful. Metaraminol (1 mg) is generally sufficient to restore coronary perfusion and a satisfactory output.

Left atrial pressure monitoring is less rewarding than in patients with chronic valve disease. The left ventricular end-diastolic pressure and the left atrial pressure rise rapidly during an attack of anginal pain; this lability of the left atrial pressure is also common during cardiac surgery and makes the management of transfusion difficult. As a general rule, the right atrial pressure is more consistent than the left, but the latter must be watched too because pulmonary oedema will occur if the left atrial pressure rises unduly. Sometimes left atrial hypertension is caused by functional mitral regurgitation; a small dose of isoprenaline may restore tone to the myocardium and eliminate regurgitation by decreasing the diameter of the mitral valve ring.

Another cause of sudden changes in left atrial pressure and in myocardial performance in the later stages of operation is mechanical disturbance to the vein graft while haemostasis is being secured. Alternatively, thrombosis can occur in the graft when protamine is given if blood flow through the vein is poor. Severe circulatory failure or cardiac arrest may follow, and it is then necessary to re-establish cardiopulmonary bypass while the graft is disobliterated.

Dysrhythmias are sometimes a notable feature of coronary arterial surgery, and there is some evidence that the incidence of both rhythm disturbances and of myocardial infarction can be decreased by heavy sedation, combined if necessary with prolonged artificial ventilation. Methoxyflurane has been advocated as an adjunct to nitrous oxide anaesthesia because of its excellent analgesic and sedative properties and possibly a specific anti-dysrhythmic effect. β-adrenergic blocking drugs are sometimes given prophylactically after perfusion has been discontinued, but this manœuvre is only safe when myocardial function is excellent. The controversy surrounding whether or not β-adrenergic blocking agents should be withdrawn before coronary arterial surgery has been discussed on p. 21.

Resection of left ventricular aneurysm

Previous myocardial infarction is the usual cause of a ventricular aneurysm. Blood clot often forms within the aneurysmal sac, and systemic embolism results, even in patients maintained on anticoagulants. The aneurysmal sac moves paradoxically during ventricular systole, and the contractile force of the rest of the ventricular muscle is dissipated in the sac so that the cardiac output falls. Resection of the aneurysm may relieve intractable cardiac failure as well as eliminate the source of embolism, but unless the residual ventricular muscle is healthy and the left ventricular cavity is of adequate size, it may be impossible to restore satisfactory function, even when the ventricular fibres are maximally stretched by a high filling pressure. Circulatory support is commonly required and may need to be continued into the postoperative period.

CONGENITAL HEART DISEASE

Some patients with congenital heart disease present in infancy. Conditions which are usually corrected at an early age are described in Chapter 9. Those which require surgery in later childhood or in adult life are described in this chapter, and only the special features which relate to infants are mentioned in Chapter 9.

Closure of secundum atrial septal defect

Patients with a secundum atrial septal defect are usually symptom free for a number of years and surgical closure in childhood or early adult life carries a very low mortality. In these uncomplicated cases, premedication, induction of anaesthesia and management before bypass are straightforward. Atrial dysrhythmias are common while the heart is being cannulated, but although the blood pressure may fall it is rare for this to give rise to concern. The defect is repaired through an incision in the right atrium; no patch is required, the ventricles are neither incised nor disturbed, and the repair is usually complete within a matter of minutes. The only hazard is that air embolism can occur if the left heart is not full of blood when the last stitch is tied in the septum. Attempts at spontaneous ventilation are often seen at this time but are no more than distracting, provided air is not sucked into a beating heart. It is usual to either clamp the aorta or induce ventricular fibrillation while the repair is in progress so that all hazard of air embolism can be eliminated. Once the atrial incision has been closed and the heart defibrillated if necessary, good function is usually restored immediately. There is rarely any need to increase the atrial pressures outside the normal range, and indeed there is a risk of causing pulmonary oedema if the heart is overfilled. The right ventricle is acclimatised to an extra volume load, and right ventricular function is so good that a high output can be generated when the right atrial pressure is normal or low. If the blood volume and hence the right atrial pressure are elevated, the output will rise even further and the corresponding left atrial pressure may be high enough to cause pulmonary oedema.

A few patients develop supraventricular dysrhythmias, particularly nodal tachycardia, in the postperfusion period. Synchronous DC defibrillation is often successful, or alternatively the rate can be controlled with digitalis. Unless dysrhythmias occur, both pulmonary and cardiac function are often so good at the end of operation that it is safe to reverse the action of muscle relaxants and restore spontaneous ventilation in young patients who have no pulmonary vascular disease.

If the defect remains uncorrected, complications are likely to occur in middle life. These include the onset of atrial fibrillation, pulmonary vascular disease which is usually associated with chronic bronchitis and airways

Table 7.1 Haemodynamic findings in a female of 57 years with the Eisenmenger syndrome complicating an ostium secundum atrial septal defect. There is pulmonary arterial hypertension with an elevated pulmonary vascular resistance. The pressure measurements are referred to zero at the mid-axillary line.

Mean right atrium	3 mm Hg (0·4 kPa)
Right ventricle	45/5 mm Hg (6/0·7 kPa)
Pulmonary artery	50/20 mm Hg (6·7/2·7 kPa)
Mean pulmonary artery	35 mm Hg (4·7 kPa)
Pulmonary arterial 'wedge'	15 mm Hg mean (2·0 kPa)
Pulmonary blood flow index	2·4 l min^{-1} m^{-2}
Pulmonary vascular resistance	5·9 units (8·3 units × m^2)
Saturation of aortic blood	80%

Table 7.2 The results of lung function testing in the same patient. There is airways obstruction, overinflation and reduced gas transfer.

	Predicted	Result
Forced expiratory volume in one second (ml)	2200	7.00
Forced vital capacity (ml)	2870	2050
Total lung capacity (ml)	4520	7710
Carbon monoxide transfer factor $(mmol\,min^{-1}\,kPa^{-1})$	5·1	3·4

obstruction, right ventricular failure, or reversal of the direction of blood flow through the defect (Eisenmenger syndrome). The latter reflects such extreme elevation of the pulmonary vascular resistance that it exceeds the systemic vascular resistance. Paradoxical embolism occurs in a few cases and reversal of blood flow through the shunt can develop acutely as a consequence of pulmonary embolism.

The condition is inoperable if the pulmonary vascular resistance is so high that flow through the defect is predominantly from right to left. When the pulmonary vascular resistance is elevated but flow is still predominantly from left to right, surgical closure is indicated; however, right ventricular failure may be troublesome in the postperfusion period, dysrhythmias are common, particularly atrial fibrillation, and many of these patients develop respiratory complications postoperatively.

Partial anomalous pulmonary venous drainage is an anomaly with physiological consequences which resemble those of a secundum atrial septal defect. One or more of the pulmonary veins enters the right atrium or superior vena cava, so causing a left to right shunt and pulmonary plethora. A patch is used to deflect blood from the pulmonary veins into the left atrium, but a single small vessel draining high into the superior vena cava is difficult to reach and can be left with safety. Total anomalous pulmonary venous drainage is a life-threatening condition which presents in infancy and is described on p. 178.

Closure of an ostium primum septal defect

The defect is low in the atrial septum, and the atrioventricular valves are often anatomically abnormal too. Functional disturbances, usually mitral regurgitation, may be present but rarely cause symptoms unless valvular incompetence is severe.

It is generally necessary to repair the defect with a patch of pericardium or of synthetic fabric, and suture or plication of the cusps or rings of the atrioventricular valves may be needed too.

The atrioventricular node is close to the site of suturing, and conduction defects occur if the node is damaged. The appearance of heart block is sometimes delayed until the postoperative period, possibly indicating oedema around the node. Postoperative management can also be complicated by residual mitral or tricuspid valve regurgitation which persists because of the abnormal shape of the valves.

Closure of ventricular septal defect

Patients with a small congenital ventricular septal defect are usually symptom free, but operative correction is more hazardous than closure of an atrial septal defect. Some form of patch is required, and most surgeons repair the

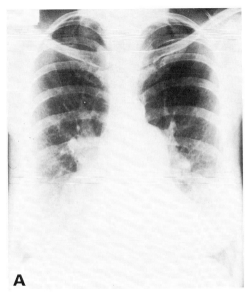

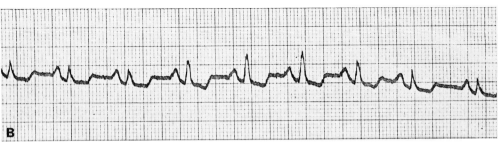

Figure 7.4 Chest X-ray and ECG of the patient described in Tables 7.1 and 7.2
  A. There is cardiomegaly, dilatation of the main pulmonary arteries and 'pruning' of peripheral vessels;
  B. ECG from standard lead II.

defect through a right ventriculotomy. Heart block can occur if the patch is secured near the atrioventricular node, and right ventricular failure is fairly common postoperatively. Patients with a large ventricular septal defect often present in infancy and require early closure or pulmonary arterial banding (p. 173). If a large defect is not closed, changes occur in the pulmonary vasculature which lead to an increase in pulmonary vascular resistance, ultimately causing reversal of the direction of blood flow through the septal defect (Eisenmenger syndrome). Gross elevation of the pulmonary vascular resistance precludes surgery, but if the pulmonary arterial pressure falls when 100% oxygen is inhaled, closure can be attempted. There is a high incidence of postoperative respiratory disturbances in patients with an elevated pulmonary vascular resistance and also in those with severe pulmonary engorgement preoperatively.

A ventricular septal defect can be acquired, usually as a result of septal rupture complicating myocardial infarction, but occasionally following trauma. Repair of a ruptured ventricular septum after myocardial infarction is particularly hazardous because the cardiac output is poor, pulmonary oedema is almost always present and the ventricular muscle is soft and friable.

Relief of pulmonary stenosis

Isolated pulmonary stenosis is a defect of the pulmonary valve, but the right ventricular muscle can become so hypertrophied that the outflow tract or infundibulum is also narrowed and contributes to the obstruction. An atrial or ventricular septal defect is sometimes present too, the direction of blood flow through it depending on the relative pressure on the two sides of the heart.

Pulmonary valvotomy can be carried out as a closed procedure, but this is rarely undertaken now because greater precision is possible if the valve is exposed. Simple valvotomy can be performed through an incision in the pulmonary artery, but a right ventricular incision is used if it is necessary to resect hypertrophied infundibular muscle. The right ventricular pressure rarely falls to normal following pulmonary valvotomy, and blood flow from right to left through an intracardiac shunt is favoured if the right-sided pressures exceed those in the left heart. A septal defect or patent foramen ovale should be sought if there is unexpected arterial hypoxaemia following relief of pulmonary stenosis.

Correction of the tetralogy of Fallot

The tetralogy consists of a high ventricular septal defect with obstruction to the outflow tract of the right ventricle. The right ventricle is hypertrophied and the origin of the aorta 'overrides' the septal defect. These patients are cyanosed from birth and develop secondary polycythaemia and its consequences (p. 18). Attacks of increased cyanosis, pallor and syncope are common in severe cases; they are caused by infundibular spasm which lowers the cardiac output and deflects a greater proportion of desaturated blood through the septal defect into the systemic circulation. Attacks can be provoked by anxiety, exercise or by inotropic drugs and can be relieved by sedation, in particular with narcotic analgesics, or by β-adrenergic blocking agents. Adoption of the 'squatting' posture is said to be a physiological response to episodes of increased outflow tract obstruction because it improves the return of blood to the right heart.

Generous premedication is essential for patients with the tetralogy of Fallot. Although severely cyanosed, they are not suffering from respiratory depression or pulmonary disease and the usual doses of narcotic analgesic drugs will not augment hypoxaemia. There is a theoretical risk of lowering the systemic vascular resistance and hence increasing the flow of blood from right to left through the septal defect, but changes in systemic vascular resistance are generally of less significance than the increase in infundibular tone which can be caused by pain, fear or crying. Furthermore, narcotic analgesics rarely cause systemic hypotension in children or young adults, and it is in these age groups that total correction of the tetralogy of Fallot is undertaken most commonly.

Anaesthesia can be induced intravenously, but cyclopropane is the agent of choice for frightened or restless children. Induction is rapid and cyclopropane decreases the tone of the infundibulum and so prevents or relieves cyanosis and circulatory disturbances induced by fear. Controlled ventilation is established in the usual way, and although the elevation of intrathoracic pressure might be expected to increase the resistance to blood flow through the lungs and hence accentuate arterial hypoxaemia, this is only the case if excessive pressures are used—perhaps because the tone of the outflow tract is lowered by anaesthesia. Hypotension and cyanosis are more likely to occur after the chest has been opened and while the heart is being handled; sometimes it is necessary to give a systemic vasopressor before the preparations for bypass have been completed.

Haemorrhage can be troublesome at this stage, particularly in patients who have had previous surgery, e.g. the 'first stage' operation of pulmonary valvotomy. Further difficulties are introduced if a palliative shunt between the systemic and pulmonary circulations has been performed in infancy and is still patent. It must be isolated and secured before bypass is established to prevent blood flowing through this low resistance pathway into the pulmonary circulation, so lowering the systemic arterial pressure and producing dangerous pulmonary congestion. It is particularly difficult to control a Potts' anastomosis between the descending aorta and left pulmonary artery. Even when surgically created shunts have been controlled, hypotension and an increase in pulmonary blood flow are common at the onset of bypass because there are extensive bronchopulmonary collateral vessels.

Complete heart block can follow total correction of the tetralogy of Fallot if the atrioventricular node or fibres of the bundle of His are damaged while the ventricular septal defect is being repaired. It is desirable to keep the heart beating while the patch is inserted, and the ECG should be watched carefully as each stitch is tied down.

Problems are common in the postperfusion period. It is often difficult to relieve right ventricular outflow tract obstruction completely, even when the infundibular muscle has been resected widely, and it may be necessary to insert a gusset to enlarge the pulmonary valve ring and root of the pulmonary artery. This results in pulmonary valve incompetence which is usually regarded as a haemodynamically unimportant lesion. Sometimes a persistently high right ventricular pressure reflects lack of development of the pulmonary vasculature which is not amenable to surgical correction, and right ventricular failure is common whenever there is any residual obstruction in the outflow tract or pulmonary circulation. Aberrant coronary vessels are often present, and further impairment of myocardial function results if these are damaged or divided during ventriculotomy.

The left ventricle is small and may be inadequate to sustain a satisfactory flow through the systemic circulation without the added thrust of the right ventricle which was previously delivering blood into the aorta too. The left atrial pressure rises, and pulmonary oedema occurs easily because the pulmonary vessels are not acclimatised to perfusion at normal volumes and pressures. The onset of severe pulmonary oedema can also signify that the ventricular septal defect has reopened.

The haemodynamic disturbances which follow total correction of the tetralogy of Fallot cannot be predicted, and it is therefore particularly necessary to monitor both atrial pressures. Transfusion requirements are guided by the higher of the two. This is usually the right atrial pressure, and values of 20 mm Hg (2·66 kPa) relative to the mid-axillary line may be needed to generate a satisfactory output. When the systemic venous pressure is so high, tricuspid incompetence is common and impedes the interpretation of the right atrial pressure. Oedema accumulates in the face, the retroperitoneal tissues and the gut, the haematocrit rises, and the cardiac output falls further because the elevated viscosity increases resistance to blood flow. Plasma rather than whole blood should be transfused if this occurs. Fresh blood or fresh frozen plasma may be needed to correct coagulation defects related to secondary polycythaemia, and the metabolic acidosis which is usually present preoperatively and often persists in the postperfusion period may require treatment.

Glenn procedure for the relief of tricuspid atresia

These patients are always cyanosed because a right to left shunt is an inevitable concomitant of tricuspid atresia. The right ventricle is rudimentary and the lungs are supplied with mixed systemic and pulmonary venous blood from the left ventricle.

The Glenn procedure is a palliative operation in which the superior vena cava is anastomosed to the right pulmonary artery. The root of the right pulmonary artery and the distal end of the superior vena cava are ligated, and therefore the superior vena caval pressure no longer reflects the filling pressure of the heart. The pressure in the superior vena cava is high postoperatively, and the patient must be nursed head-up to diminish cerebral oedema. The combination of a high caval pressure, polycythaemia, and vascular damage at the site of the anastomosis favours cerebral venous thrombosis. Further damage to the great veins must be avoided at all costs; intravenous infusion and monitoring lines must never be placed in the jugular, subclavian or innominate veins, and it is preferable to avoid cannulating any vein which drains into the superior vena cava.

The same constraints apply if a superior caval-pulmonary arterial anastomosis is constructed as part of the Fontan procedure, an operation which is used to achieve some degree of physiological correction for tricuspid atresia. As well as redirecting superior caval blood into the right pulmonary artery, a valved-conduit is inserted to carry blood from the inferior vena cava or right atrium to the left pulmonary artery. The root of the main pulmonary artery is then ligated.

EMERGENCY OPEN HEART SURGERY

Emergency open heart surgery is only undertaken to relieve immediately life-threatening cardiac disease. Common indications are pulmonary embolectomy in patients who are unsuitable for treatment with streptokinase (p. 127), and critical obstruction or regurgitation affecting one or more valves. Sudden deterioration can be caused by dehiscence of a prosthetic valve or thrombosis on its surface, by perforation of a valve cusp as a complication of subacute bacterial endocarditis, or by impaction of a left atrial myxoma in the orifice of the mitral valve. Occasionally, an aortic dissection extending to the ascending aorta and aortic valve requires urgent surgery; myocardial trauma, and ventricular septal rupture or intractable dysrhythmias associated with myocardial infarction account for a tiny percentage of emergency cases.

These patients are almost always unprepared and assessment is often incomplete. Signs of circulatory failure are usually present, some patients are already intubated and maintained on intermittent positive pressure ventila-

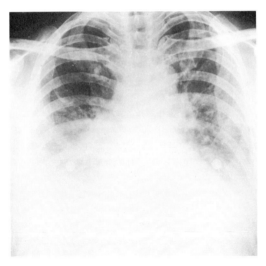

Figure 7.5 Emergency mitral valve replacement: male aged 71. Successful operation followed six weeks' deteriorating left ventricular failure caused by chordal rupture and mitral incompetence complicating myocardial infarction.
Preoperative chest X-ray.

Table 7.3 Haemodynamic findings in the same patient (pressure measurements referred to zero at the mid-axillary line).

Mean right atrium	12 mm Hg (1·6 kPa)
Right ventricle	70/8 mm Hg (8·3/1·1 kPa)
Right ventricular end-diastolic	12 mm Hg (1·6 kPa)
Pulmonary artery	70/35 mm Hg (8·3/4·7 kPa)
Left ventricle	100/15 mm Hg (13·3/2·0 kPa)
Left ventricular end-diastolic	25 mm Hg (3·3 kPa)
Mixed venous oxygen saturation	32%
The pulmonary arterial 'wedge' position was not reached.	

tion, and in the majority, consciousness is sufficiently obtunded for control of anxiety to be relatively unimportant. Premedication should therefore be minimal—either no premedication or a small dose of atropine or hyoscine is sufficient. Whenever possible, arterial and venous cannulae should be inserted and pressure monitoring established before anaesthesia is induced. Similarly, drugs required for resuscitation should be prepared beforehand, and the usual precautions for dealing with the full stomach must be available.

Cannulation of the femoral vessels under local anaesthesia followed by femoro-femoral bypass (femoral vein to femoral artery), has been advocated as a means of providing circulatory support during the induction of anaesthesia and while the heart is being cannulated. However, this technique introduces delay and most experienced teams prefer to proceed immediately without extracorporeal support.

Spontaneously breathing patients are preoxygenated, but an inhalational induction is contraindicated because of the risks of hypoxaemia (nitrous oxide), hypotension (halothane), or an increase in pulmonary vascular resistance (cyclopropane). Intravenous diazepam ($0.1–0.5$ mg/kg) is a useful agent for inducing anaesthesia without adding to the circulatory disturbances; alternatively, a small dose of thiopentone ($0.3–1$ mg/kg) is usually safe. After intubation, anaesthesia is continued with nitrous oxide and oxygen, using higher than normal concentrations of oxygen if necessary. Many of these patients are so sick that an adequate depth of anaesthesia can be maintained with controlled ventilation and 50% nitrous oxide in oxygen but a few require additional analgesia. Narcotic drugs must be given in very small increments because patients requiring emergency cardiac surgery are vasoconstricted, and unacceptable degrees of hypotension occur very readily if arterial tone is reduced. Inotropic or vasopressor agents are often needed between induction and the start of bypass, but circulatory function can improve dramatically in the postperfusion period if the haemodynamic abnormality has been corrected completely. Whenever there has been a prolonged period of circulatory insufficiency, renal function should be monitored with particular care, and metabolic acidosis and electrolyte disturbances should be sought and treated.

Pulmonary embolectomy

The current treatment for massive pulmonary embolism is infusion of streptokinase into the pulmonary artery. Haemodynamic improvement can be detected after about 6 hours and the infusion is generally continued for 36 hours to 3 days. The chief side-effect is haemorrhage, and streptokinase is contraindicated in patients already at risk from haemorrhage, e.g. those recovering from very recent surgery, or suffering from active peptic ulceration. Streptokinase is also contraindicated in patients who have already had a cardiac arrest caused by pulmonary embolism or who are moribund and unlikely to survive the 6 hours needed before haemodynamic improvement can be expected.

These patients require pulmonary embolectomy. The problems which they present always include acute circulatory failure and arterial hypoxaemia; anuria is common and many will have been given anticoagulants, either heparin or streptokinase. Some have suffered a cardiac arrest and have neurological damage as a result, and in a few cases the predisposing condition may influence anaesthetic management (e.g. recent orthopaedic surgery).

The principles outlined in the preceding section on anaesthesia for emergency open heart surgery all apply. It is particularly important to avoid induction with cyclopropane and oxygen because cardiac arrest can easily follow the increase in pulmonary vascular resistance which occurs. This action of cyclopropane is notable because it is so different from its effect on the outflow tract of the right ventricle (p. 123).

Features of management which are specific to patients requiring pulmonary embolectomy are the choice of methods of circulatory support and the management of anticoagulants.

Circulatory failure in pulmonary embolism is caused by abrupt occlusion of a large percentage of the pulmonary vascular bed. A previously normal right ventricle is unable to generate sufficient pressure to overcome this obstruction, little blood reaches the left heart and the cardiac output falls. Initially, left ventricular function is undisturbed, but it too deteriorates when the low output state has been present for some time. However, the left atrial pressure remains lower than that on the right and pulmonary oedema cannot be generated in the usual way, although it can occur when flow is restored to a previously occluded subdivision of the pulmonary vascular bed.

A high right atrial pressure is essential to maintain right ventricular filling, but in the most severe cases the right ventricle is so grossly overdistended that its limited output is independent of changes in filling pressure. Patients without gross elevation of the right atrial and right ventricular end-diastolic pressure may therefore be improved by transfusion, but those in whom these pressures are already very high are uninfluenced or deteriorate if transfused (deterioration probably indicating an increase in tricuspid incompetence).

Inotropic agents can be used to improve right ventricular function. Isoprenaline not only increases the force of myocardial contraction but also lowers the pulmonary vascular resistance and may therefore relieve obstruction caused by pulmonary arterial spasm in vessels which are not occluded by the embolus. The disadvantage of isoprenaline is that it lowers the diastolic pressure in systemic arteries which may decrease coronary flow to the right ventricle. Deterioration following isoprenaline has been documented in experimental pulmonary embolism in dogs, but in man, haemodynamic improvement can often be demonstrated.

It is sometimes argued that vasopressor drugs are preferable to isoprenaline because they increase the systemic vascular resistance and improve coronary perfusion. The increase in left ventricular after-load is regarded as unimportant because it is the right ventricle and not the left which is requiring most support. Infusions of metaraminol are chosen if an increase in diastolic pressure is required, but the disadvantage of this drug is that it increases the pulmonary vascular resistance too and adds to the already elevated after-load on the right ventricle. The combined α- and β-adrenergic stimulant properties of adrenaline may be preferable; although the diastolic pressure in the systemic vessels tends to fall in normal subjects, the increase in output which results when adrenaline is given to patients with circulatory failure is such

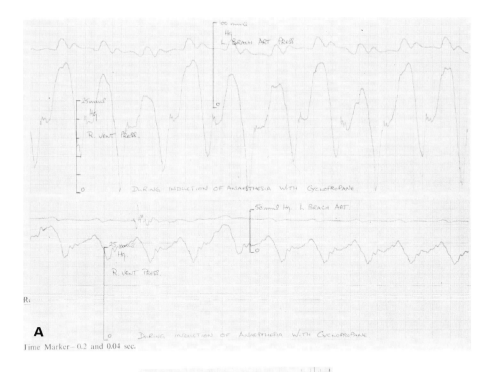

Time Marker—0.2 and 0.04 sec.

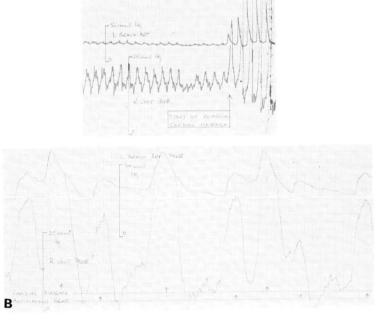

Figure 7.6 Arterial and right ventricular pressure records, referred to zero at the sternal angle, obtained during the induction of anaesthesia with cyclopropane in a patient suffering from massive pulmonary embolism. The right ventricular end-diastolic pressure was elevated (12 mm Hg; 1·6 kPa) before induction and rose progressively until cardiac arrest occurred. External cardiac massage emptied the heart and a spontaneous heart beat was restored.

A, during induction of anaesthesia; B, Successful cardiac massage.

Reproduced by courtesy of Dr. R. D. Bradley, St. Thomas' Hospital.

that both systolic and diastolic pressure usually rise. Similarly, in patients with pulmonary embolism, the inotropic effect on the right ventricle is more prominent that any increase in pulmonary vascular resistance. If the circulation cannot be supported with adrenaline, intermittent injections of calcium chloride (2–5 mmol) may just keep the heart beating until it is possible to institute cardiopulmonary bypass. With this degree of circulatory failure, heparin may not mix effectively with the entire blood volume, and a few moments of cardiac massage after it is injected help to prevent obstruction to the extracorporeal circuit by blood clot.

Some patients requiring emergency pulmonary embolectomy will have been given heparin already. In the circumstances of extreme circulatory failure outlined above, this is nothing but an asset. In spite of pretreatment with heparin, it is customary to give the usual dose immediately before bypass and rarely necessary to use more than the normal quantities of protamine afterwards. Pretreatment with streptokinase is less hazardous than might be anticipated. The effect is short-lived, and if the infusion is discontinued when the decision to operate is taken, abnormal bleeding is rarely a problem. Attempts to reverse the effects of streptokinase with antifibrinolytic drugs are unnecessary, and if haemorrhage does appear excessive, it can be controlled with fresh frozen plasma.

It is generally possible to clear the entire pulmonary vascular bed during bypass. An incision is made in the main pulmonary artery, large clots are removed and smaller fragments are eliminated from the distal vessels by suction combined with gentle artificial ventilation. Ultimately there should be free bleeding into the pulmonary arterial incision from all the visible subdivisions, blood reaching the left heart through thebesian veins and bronchial vessels. In spite of the parlous condition of these patients preoperatively, the results of surgery are excellent provided cardiac arrest can be avoided before bypass is established.

REFERENCES

CHRONIC VALVE DISEASE

BAXTER R. H., BAIN W. H., RANKIN R. J., TURNER R. A., ESCAROUS E. A., THOMSON R. M., LORIMER A. R. & LAWRIE T. D. V. (1975) Tricuspid valve replacement: a five year appraisal. *Thorax* **30**, 158.

CAVES P. K. & PANETH M. (1973) Non-rheumatic 'subvalvar' mitral regurgitation. *Thorax* **28**, 158.

EFFLER D. B. (1975) Do prosthetic heart valves really make clots? *Journal of Thoracic and Cardiovascular Surgery* **69**, 664.

IONESCU M. I., PAKRASHI B. C., MARY D. A. S., BARTEK I. T. & WOOLER G. H. (1974) Long term evaluation of tissue valves. *Journal of Thoracic and Cardiovascular Surgery* **68**, 361.

Ross D. N., & Parker J. D. (1974) Current aspects of valve replacement. In *Progress in Cardiology*, Ed. P. N. Yu & J. F. Goodwin, p. 253. Lea & Febiger, Philadelphia.

Wisheart J. D., Ross D. N. & Ross J. K. (1972) A review of the effect of previous operations on the results of open heart surgery. *Thorax* **27**, 137.

ISCHAEMIC HEART DISEASE

Cleland W. P. (1976) The role of surgery in coronary artery disease. *Postgraduate Medical Journal* **52**, 462.

Gerbode F., Kerth W. J., Hill J. D., Banerjee S. & Marcelletti C. (1974) Elective operation for left ventricular asynergy. *Thorax* **29**, 282.

Julian D. G. (1975) Aorta to coronary bypass surgery for angina. In *Modern Trends in Cardiology* 3, Ed. M. F. Oliver, p. 439. Butterworth, London.

Leading Article (1974) Aorto-coronary bypass grafting for angina. *British Medical Journal* **4**, 61.

Lewis B. S. & Gotsman M. S. (1974) Sudden death in patients awaiting coronary artery surgery. *Thorax* **29**, 209.

Mundth E. D. & Austen W. G. (1975) Surgical measures for coronary heart disease. *New England Journal of Medicine* **293**, pp. 13, 75, 124.

Redondo J., Novakovic L., Olivari F. & Penna M. (1971) The effects of methoxyflurane on myocardial contractility and reactivity. *Anesthesiology* **34**, 450.

Rowe G. G. (1974) Responses of the coronary circulation to physiologic changes and pharmacologic agents. *Anesthesiology* **41**, 182.

Sbokos C. G., Monro J. L. Ross J. K. (1976) Elective operations for post-infarction left ventricular aneurysms. *Thorax* **31**,55.

Viljoen J. F., Estafanous F. G. & Kim K. S. (1974) Anaesthesia for emergency coronary artery surgery. *British Journal of Anaesthesia* **46**, 953.

Wynands J. E., Sheridan C. A., Batra M. S., Palmer W. H. & Shanks J. (1970) Coronary artery disease. *Anesthesiology* **33**, 260.

CONGENITAL HEART DISEASE

Daniel F. J., Clarke C. P., Richardson J. P., Westlake G. W. & Jones P. G. (1976) An evaluation of Potts' aortopulmonary shunt for palliation of cyanotic heart disease. *Thorax* **31**, 394.

Flamm M. D., Cohn K. E. & Hancock E. W. (1970) Ventricular function in atrial septal defect. *American Journal of Medicine* **48**, 286.

Knight M. & Lennox S. (1972) Results of surgery for atrial septal defect in patients of 40 years and over. *Thorax* **27**, 577.

Matthews H. R. & Belsey R. H. R. (1973) Indications for the Brock operation in current treatment of tetralogy of Fallot. *Thorax* **28**, 1.

Prusty S. & Ross D. N. (1975) Adult cyanotic congenital heart disease. *Thorax* **30**, 650.

Reid J. M., Coleman E. N., Barclay R. S. & Stevenson J. G. (1973) Blalock–Taussig anastomosis in 126 patients with Fallot's tetralogy. *Thorax* **28**, 269.

EMERGENCY OPEN HEART SURGERY

Beall A. C. & Collins J. J. (1975) Editorial: what is the role of pulmonary embolectomy? *American Heart Journal* **89**, 411.

Miller M. G., Weintraub R. G., Hedley–White J., Restall D. S. & Alexander M. (1974) Surgery for cardiogenic shock. *Lancet* **2**, 1342.

PRICE H. L., COOPERMAN L. H., WARDEN J. C., MORRIS J. J. & SMITH T. C. (1969) Pulmonary hemodynamics during general anesthesia in man. *Anesthesiology* **30,** 629.

ROSENBERG J. C., HUSSAIN R. & LENAGHAN R. (1971) Isoproterenol and norepinephrine therapy for pulmonary embolism shock. *Journal of Thoracic and Cardiovascular Surgery* **62,** 144.

SASAHARA A. A. (1974) Therapy for pulmonary embolism. *Journal of the American Medical Association* **229,** 1795.

SASAHARA A. A. (1974) Current problems in pulmonary embolism: introduction. *Progress in Cardiovascular Diseases* **17,** 161.

SAUTTER R. D., MYERS W. O., RAY J. F. 3rd & WENZEL F. J. (1975) Pulmonary embolectomy: review and current status. *Progress in Cardiovascular Diseases* **17,** 371.

CHAPTER 8

EXTRACORPOREAL CIRCULATION AND ASSOCIATED TECHNIQUES

The scope of early attempts at cardiac surgery was limited by the need to preserve effective heart action throughout the operation. During the early 1950's, several techniques were developed to circumvent this need.

A few patients with congenital heart disease were operated on with circulatory support provided by a close, haematologically compatible relative, generally a parent. The technique was never widely used because it was unsuitable for adult patients and hazards to the supporting partner posed a number of ethical difficulties.

The introduction of systemic hypothermia marked an important advance. Tissue oxygen requirements fall to approximately 70% of basal at 30°C, and periods of ischaemia which would be lethal at normal temperatures can be tolerated without apparent harm. Surface cooling to this temperature can be achieved by immersing the anaesthetised patient in a bath of iced water or by covering the body with wet sheets and creating a wind tunnel with fans. Gastric lavage with iced saline has also been used. When cooling has been discontinued, the chest is opened, the cavae are snared and the aorta is clamped. Simple procedures such as repair of a secundum atrial septal defect or relief of isolated pulmonary stenosis can then be carried out in the 10-minute period of circulatory arrest which is generally regarded as safe at this temperature. The patient is rewarmed postoperatively, either by immersion in warm water or by using heated blankets.

Cerebral damage is common if the circulation is arrested for much more than 10 minutes. The chief hazard however is ventricular fibrillation induced by cooling. This can occur before the chest has been opened or, more commonly, when the heart is handled. It is particularly dangerous in these circumstances because the heart is too cold to defibrillate easily and cannot be rewarmed quickly. Hypothermia induced by venovenous cooling is an alternative technique which provides slightly better temperature control. The cavae are cannulated and blood is pumped from one to the other through a heat exchanger. Body temperature can be changed more rapidly than with surface cooling but the duration of circulatory arrest is still limited to 10 minutes, and rewarming cannot be achieved easily if the heart fibrillates.

Further progress awaited the development of extracorporeal oxygenators which were introduced into clinical practice in the 1950's, and it is possible now to maintain satisfactory perfusion for prolonged periods while the heart is excluded from the systemic circulation. A brief outline of the modern technique of cardiopulmonary bypass has been given in Chapter 6. Aspects of the extracorporeal system are considered in greater detail here.

COLLECTION AND RETURN OF BLOOD TO THE PATIENT

Venous drainage

Systemic venous blood is returned to the oxygenator through two flexible plastic cannulae which are inserted into the superior and inferior venae cavae through separate right atrial incisions, and then joined to create a single drainage channel. Alternatively, a single cannula is placed in the right atrium. Blood flows freely into the oxygenator under the influence of gravity, provided the operating table is high enough and there is no 'air lock' caused by bubbles trapped in the tubing when it is joined to the cannulae. Mechanical suction to encourage drainage is undesirable because the negative pressure may entrain air or may suck the walls of the cavae against the orifices of the cannulae. The venous pressures distal to the sites of cannulation should be low, even after snares have been tightened around the cavae and their contained cannulae; any elevation of the venous pressures suggests mechanical obstruction which should be sought and corrected. This is particularly necessary if the superior caval pressure is high because the cerebral blood flow is jeopardised if the perfusion pressure (mean arterial minus mean venous pressure) is low. If the venous pressures remain elevated, oedema will accumulate and

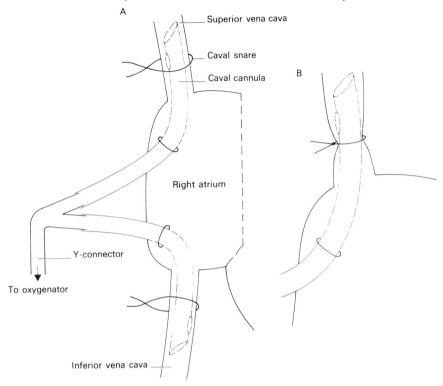

A

Superior vena cava

Caval snare

Caval cannula

B

Right atrium

Y-connector

To oxygenator

Inferior vena cava

Figure 8.1   Schematic diagrams to illustrate the siting of caval cannulae during A, partial and B, total cardiopulmonary bypass.

capillary damage will occur, so causing bleeding into the tissues which is obvious postoperatively as petechiae on the chest wall or subconjunctival haemorrhages. Obstruction to the venous drainage is much less likely to occur if a single fenestrated right atrial cannula is used, but this can only be chosen when the right heart will not be opened because some venous blood will enter the right atrium and obscure the surgical field.

Intracardiac suction

The heart does not empty completely, even when the caval cannulae are in place and the snares are secured. The coronary sinus enters the right atrium separately, a number of unnamed vessels enter both atria, and there is also a considerable volume of blood within the cavities of a distended heart. Hand-held suckers are used to return this blood to the oxygenator and to keep the surgical field dry, but blood which is contaminated with clot or debris from the heart or pericardial cavity should be discarded. The intracardiac suckers should be used as little as possible because haemolysis occurs when a mixture of blood and air is exposed to a negative pressure, and suction near the coronary sinus should be avoided altogether because the cardiac conducting tissue can be damaged there.

Left ventricular vent

If blood returns to the left side of the heart when the cavities are intact but the heart is not beating, the pressure will rise in both the left ventricle and left atrium. This damages the left ventricular muscle, distends the mitral valve ring, and generates excessive pressure in the pulmonary capillaries which is manifest as pulmonary oedema or haemorrhage either during bypass or immediately afterwards.

Undesirable left ventricular distension is eliminated by using a separate drainage tube or vent. This is usually introduced through the apex of the ventricle but can be inserted through the left atrium and mitral valve if the left ventricular muscle is too friable, or if there are adhesions which prevent easy access to the apex. Other uses of the vent are to ensure a bloodless field (e.g. during surgery on the aortic valve), to provide a route for eliminating air from the left heart when surgery is complete, and finally, to act as an 'overflow' when the heart is beating but is too feeble to eject efficiently through the aortic valve. Suction may not be required to prevent overdistension but must be available to control aortic incompetence, or if a completely bloodless field is required within the left heart.

Blood returned through the vent and intracardiac suckers passes through a filter and defoaming unit before it enters the oxygenator, and a reservoir is often included in the circuit at this site to accommodate the large volume of blood which may be encountered when the heart is first opened.

Arterial return

Oxygenated blood is returned to the patient through a cannula in either the ascending aorta or one femoral artery (usually the left). This is generally the narrowest part of the circuit and the cannula should be as short as possible and as large as the diameter of the vessel permits. It may be difficult to introduce a cannula of adequate size if the femoral artery is small or atheromatous and the vessel wall may be damaged. If this is unrecognised at the time, dissection of the femoral artery can extend to the iliac vessels or even the aorta when bypass is established. There is also a definite postoperative morbidity associated with femoral arterial cannulation, in particular, sepsis, the formation of a false aneurysm, or the development of a lymphatic fistula.

Cannulation of the ascending aorta is generally preferred at the present time unless the aortic arch is the site of surgery. Damage to the aortic wall is rare when the cannula is inserted, but repair of the cannulation site can be difficult if the wall is thin and friable; a false aneurysm develops occasion-ally and may rupture when the sternum is reopened to repair it. If the aortic cannula becomes misplaced during perfusion, the innominate artery can be excluded from the circulation or the entire flow may be delivered through this vessel. Cerebral damage is inevitable in either circumstance but some protection is afforded if the anaesthetist confirms the presence of symmetrical pulsation in the carotid arteries after the cannula has been inserted.

Coronary perfusion

The coronary arteries are usually perfused during bypass by blood which flows in a retrograde direction from the site of cannulation to the closed aortic valve, but this supply is interrupted if the aorta is cross-clamped. Aortic cross-clamping may be necessary to control retrograde flow in the presence of aortic incompetence, to permit access to the aortic valve, to prevent air in the left ventricle reaching the cerebral circulation, or to facilitate surgery by inducing ischaemic arrest of the heart. The myocardium can recover after surprisingly long periods of ischaemia (e.g. 30 to 45 minutes) even at a normal body tem-perature, provided a good coronary flow is restored before circulatory sup-port is withdrawn. Some myocardial damage is inevitable but can be minimised during aortic valve surgery by separate cannulation and perfusion of the coronary arteries. If the aortic valve is competent and is not the site of surgery, the root of the aorta can be perfused when necessary through a cannula inserted proximal to the aortic cross-clamp, or the clamp can be re-moved intermittently for short periods.

The myocardium can be damaged if the coronary arteries are perfused at too high a pressure or with an excessive flow. If an independent coronary arterial supply is anticipated, it is preferable to arrange for this to be delivered at a known pressure through a pair of flowmeters which are calibrated from 0 to 500 ml/minute. Sometimes a separate pump is used too. The coronary cannulae can be secured in place with snares, but self-retaining cannulae are selected more commonly. These incorporate a balloon at the tip which inflates as soon as blood flows through the cannula against a slight resistance. The perfusion pressure and flow rate to the coronary system are noted, but the best index of adequate perfusion is the maintenance or restoration of a coordi-nated heart beat and a normal ECG.

Sometimes it is impossible to cannulate the coronary ostia because of ana-tomical difficulties or disease. Fragments of atheroma can be dislodged and impacted in the coronary system, the wall of the vessel may be disrupted, and the presence of the cannulae may impede access to the surgical field. For these reasons, coronary perfusion is not undertaken routinely whenever the aortic valve is to be replaced. Each case must be judged individually, but the likelihood of prolonged ischaemia in a patient with known left ventricular dysfunction is generally regarded as an indication for coronary arterial cannulation from the outset.

OXYGENATORS

Three types of oxygenators are in use at the present time.

Rotating disc oxygenators

A series of thin, stainless steel or polycarbonate discs are mounted on a spindle. The entire assembly is suspended in a cylindrical chamber which is about one-third filled with a suitable priming fluid (p. 144). Blood and fresh gas, usually 2·5% carbon dioxide in oxygen, are delivered to one end of the chamber, the former entering the reservoir of fluid and the latter passing through the gas-filled space above it. As the spindle rotates, the plates are drawn through the blood and emerge covered with a thin film of blood which equilibrates with the gaseous atmosphere of the oxygenator. The exit for arterialised blood is at the opposite end of the chamber, well below the level of the blood–gas interface. Air bubbles are generated near the surface of the blood as the discs rotate, and this layer extends more deeply as the speed of rotation increases. Some bubbles escape into the arterial supply to the patient, especially if the blood level in the oxygenator falls too low. These factors limit the performance of the system, but the oxygen transfer capacity

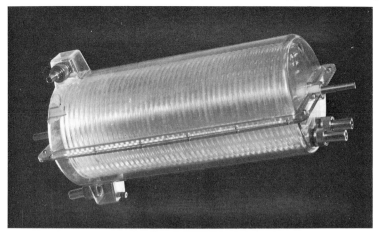

Figure 8.2 A rotating disc oxygenator for paediatric use. Venous drainage and blood returned by suction enter the oxygenator through the orifices on the lower right; the arterial return leaves the oxygenator at the lower left while gas enters through the upper left orifice and leaves through a hole in the wall of the oxygenator, visible at the right hand end.

of a large disc oxygenator with the discs rotating at 120 rpm can easily reach 250 ml/minute.

Bubble oxygenators

This term includes a number of different devices which all operate on a similar principle; many of them are made of disposable materials and are supplied presterilised.

Gas exchange occurs across the large surface area which is formed when myriads of bubbles are generated by the dispersal of a gas supply within the venous blood. These bubbles must be eliminated again before the oxygenated blood is returned to the patient, and different oxygenators differ in the design of the defoaming chamber. The performance of oxygenators of this type is usually limited by the efficiency of the defoaming chamber, and gas bubbles which can be detected by ultrasonic monitoring reach the patient through the arterial line with all these devices. In some models, the defoaming capacity is exhausted with the passage of time.

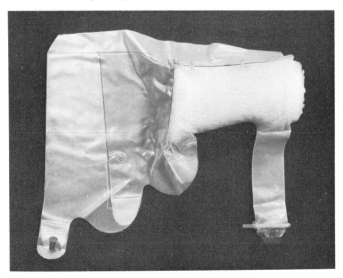

Figure 8.3 A bubble oxygenator. Blood and gas enter the chimney on the right. Defrothing takes place in the mesh at the top of the chimney, and oxygenated blood passes through the settling chambers and filters before leaving for return to the patient through the orifice at the bottom left.

Membrane oxygenators

A semipermeable membrane is closely folded in such a way that a large surface area is provided within a compact frame. Some membranes have a microporous structure.

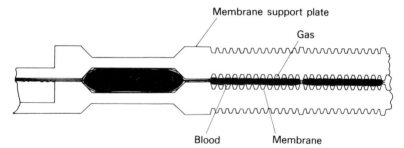

Figure 8.4 Cross-section of two plates of a Landé-Edwards membrane oxygenator showing capillaries formed by membrane and plates. Reproduced by permission of Edwards Laboratories.

Two channels are created, one being used for the passage of blood and the other for gas. Blood cannot cross the membrane, but gas exchange occurs readily without any mixing of the two phases. Blood damage and the generation of gas bubbles are minimised, and these devices are therefore used for prolonged extracorporeal support as well as during surgery. Developments are rapid in this field at the present time and are aimed at producing membrane oxygenators at low cost, in which the integrity of the membrane can be guaranteed, and in which gas exchange is adequate to support the entire requirements of a normothermic adult over a prolonged period of time. The oxygen transfer capacity of oxygenators made with a microporous Teflon membrane (pore size $1-5\,\mu$m) is between 100 and 150 ml m^{-2} min^{-1}.

ARTERIAL PUMPS

Various types of pumps have been used to return blood from the oxygenator to the patient, but the roller pump is the only design which has remained popular. Pumps with large bore tubing and slowly rotating rollers are preferred because these features minimise damage to both the blood and to the walls of the tubing. There is also less wear on the tubing if the rollers are adjusted so that they are only just occlusive. The flow rate is calculated from the stroke volume and number of revolutions per minute, but the delivered flow deviates from the theoretical value as the speed of rotation increases because the tubing fails to refill completely when it is released.

The waveform of the pressure generated by a roller pump is barely pulsatile, and there is some evidence which suggests that organ dysfunction is less likely to occur during perfusion with pumps which generate a pulsatile waveform bearing some resemblance to that seen in the normal circulation. Unfortunately, pumps of this type are difficult to construct, and very high pressure gradients develop because blood only flows intermittently through the narrow arterial cannula.

The pressure at which blood is returned to the arterial system must be monitored carefully; a large pressure gradient across the arterial cannula increases red cell destruction and favours the formation of cavitation bubbles on the low pressure side of the obstruction. When the arterial cannula is first inserted, pressure transients equal to the systemic arterial pressure should be transmitted to the manometer of the extracorporeal system. Ideally, the pressure gradient between the pump and systemic vessels should not exceed 100 mm Hg (13·3 kPa) or so once perfusion has started, but this is only possible if the arterial cannula is of adequate diameter and has been positioned satisfactorily.

TEMPERATURE CONTROL

Many oxygenators incorporate an integral heat-exchanging circuit but a separate heat exchanger is sometimes preferred. This consists of two concentric stainless steel cylinders. Blood flows through the narrow annulus between them and water at the desired temperature flows through the central chamber and around the outside. Rapid changes in temperature can be induced with some heat exchangers, performance depending on the dimensions of the device and the flow rates of both blood and water. A gradient of more than 15°C between the blood and the patient's body is undesirable because it promotes inequalities of temperature between organs perfused at different flow rates; it also encourages the formation of bubbles during rewarming when the solubility of gases is reduced. Postoperative cerebral damage has been related to overrapid cooling, and plasma proteins can be denatured if the blood temperature is allowed to reach much more than 40°C. An acceptable rate of cooling is not more than $1°C\,min^{-1}$.

FILTRATION

The need for filtration of blood returned from the cardiac cavities has been described already, but filtration is also required before blood can be delivered from the oxygenator to the patient. Platelet aggregates, fibrin strands and adherent leucocytes develop *in vivo* during episodes of circulatory stress. Normally these are removed by filtration in the lungs, but during extracorporeal circulation they are returned to the oxygenator. Similar aggregates accumulate in stored blood; these too are removed by the lungs when blood is transfused intravenously but not when it is added to the reservoir of an extracorporeal circuit. Not all the debris is derived from formed elements in the blood. Fat from the pericardial cavity, blood clot, vegetations or calcium from within the heart, and particulate material derived from the apparatus (e.g.

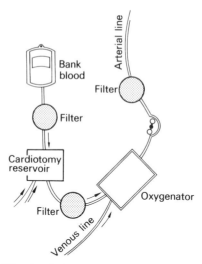

Figure 8.5 Sites of filtration during cardiopulmonary bypass, from Reed and Clark, reproduced by permission of Texas Medical Press.

antifoam) can all be identified in blood returning from the oxygenator. At one time, arterial filters consisted of a simple metal mesh, pore size 150–300 μm. It was feared that use of a finer mesh would create a site of obstruction to flow and would filter out excessive numbers of platelets. More recently, small pore filters (25–40 μm pore size) have been used to eliminate microemboli. They consist of either Dacron wool or polyester mesh, and their use is associated with both clinical and laboratory evidence of diminished embolic damage following bypass. They are, however, ineffective in removing fat emboli and may merely break up air emboli into smaller bubbles.

SELECTION AND MAINTENANCE OF PERFUSION APPARATUS

There is a great variety of extracorporeal apparatus available, and selection is often a matter of individual team preference.

The items chosen must be assembled in a circuit which eliminates sharp angles and narrow orifices where blood damage may occur or where turbulence in the blood stream might create gaseous emboli. Junctions on the high pressure side of the circuit must be secured firmly, e.g. with O-rings or with screw fittings. Unnecessary lengths of tubing should be avoided because they drag on intravascular cannulae and are liable to kink.

If reusable equipment (e.g. a rotating disc oxygenator) is chosen, staff must be available to clean and sterilise it. Metal surfaces must be checked to ensure they are smooth, fittings which screw together must be carefully matched, and the mechanical and electrical performance of all the apparatus must be checked regularly.

All parts of the circuit which come into contact with the patient's blood must be sterilised before use. Some equipment can be autoclaved and some is already sterilised by irradiation or ethylene oxide when it is supplied. Components such as circuit tubing are generally cut to length and sterilised on site.

Plastic materials which have been sterilised with ethylene oxide may contain residual ethylene oxide, or ethylene glycol which is formed in the presence of water. These substances are toxic and may be detrimental if leached out during perfusion. Equipment made from PVC may contain significant amounts of ethylene oxide, but silicone rubber retains very little. A shelf life of 21 days for sterilised items allows ethylene oxide to diffuse slowly out of the plastic, and this can be accelerated if the packs are exposed to heat and ventilation.

The entire process of selection of apparatus, its maintenance and sterilisation, and setting up and running the perfusion requires a team of highly trained technical staff.

ASSEMBLING AND PRIMING THE EXTRACORPOREAL CIRCUIT

The sterile circuit is assembled in, or close to, the operating theatre. Covers are only removed from the cut ends of tubing when each junction is ready to be completed. The system is then flushed to remove final traces of ethylene oxide residues or any particulate material trapped inside when the circuit was assembled. This is particularly necessary with some membrane oxygenators which are packed with salt crystals; dangerous hypernatraemia results unless the salt is removed entirely. Dextrose 5% is generally used to flush the circuit and a small residue (200 ml or so) may remain and form part of the priming volume.

The apparatus is now ready to be moved into the operating theatre. The ends of a loop of sterile tubing are passed from the operating table and are joined to the venous entry site on the oxygentator and to the arterial line distal to the filters. This completes an extracorporeal circuit through a loop or 'sash' and the circuit can now be primed. At the same time, the ends of additional lines which will be used for the intracardiac suction, left ventricular vent and coronary perfusion are passed to or from the table.

At one time it was customary to prime the extracorporeal circuit with whole blood but some degree of haemodilution is now used routinely. If the haematocrit is halved, the oxygen-carrying capacity of the blood is approximately halved too, but at the same time the viscosity is greatly reduced and blood flows through the microvasculature more readily. Tissue oxygenation is unimpaired and may even be improved when the haematocrit is about 30%, and satisfactory oxygen transport can still be achieved when the packed cell volume is 20%, provided a high blood flow is ensured. Lowering the haematocrit to this degree permits greater latitude in the volume of electrolyte solution used for the prime, but a high flow rate throughout perfusion is an essential part of this technique.

The extracorporeal circuit requires a total priming volume of between 1·5 and 3·0 litres depending on the choice of equipment, particularly the oxygenator. At least 30 ml/kg of electrolyte solution can be used for adult patients who are not anaemic. A mixture of 2 l of Ringer lactate solution, 1 l of 5% dextrose and 100 mmol of sodium bicarbonate solution (1 mmol/ml) provides an isotonic mixture with a sodium concentration of approximately 140 mmol/l and a pH within the physiological range. Potassium chloride can be added to the prime or is withheld until a good urinary output is established during perfusion. Potassium is then added at a rate of approximately 15 mmol/200 ml of urine passed. Some patients require considerably larger quantities to maintain the plasma concentration within the normal range.

Part of the priming volume is retained by the patient; initially it is redistributed between the various compartments of body fluids, and ultimately it is excreted, diuretic therapy being prescribed postoperatively if necessary. A large diuresis is commonly established during perfusion and an equal volume of electrolyte solution can be added to replace the urine passed. Whole blood is given to maintain the haematocrit between 20 and 30%, and is also included in the priming volume for cardiac surgery in infants, for patients who are anaemic, or for those in severe congestive cardiac failure who already have a considerable increase in extracellular fluid volume. Blood stored for prolonged periods is undesirable—it is acidotic and hyperkalaemic, the content of particulate debris increases with time, and the red cells are easily damaged by mechanical trauma. Ideally, blood required for cardiopulmonary bypass is collected into heparin on the day of operation. This can be used during bypass without further additives but must be discarded after about 24 hours because the heparin is slowly inactivated, even during refrigeration. ACD or CPD blood is used more often, but preferably should be less than 2 days old. Heparinisation and reconstitution of calcium levels are required before it can be used during perfusion. 30 mg heparin are added to each unit of 500 ml followed by 2·25 mmol of calcium chloride. If a large electrolyte load is considered undesirable but whole blood is to be avoided, the prime may contain colloidal solutions such as human plasma protein fraction, dextran or gelatin derivatives. None of these products carry a risk of homologous serum jaundice; dextran may, however, interfere with coagulation mechanisms. Heparin is occasionally added, even to a non-haem prime.

Gas supply to the oxygenator

Carbon dioxide elimination and oxygen uptake both occur in the oxygenator, but the efficiency of gas exchange is not necessarily the same for the two processes and may differ from one oxygenator to another. Hypocapnia should be avoided because it interferes with peripheral perfusion and causes cerebral vasoconstriction, and the gas mixture supplied to the oxygenator should be adjusted to maintain a normal arterial carbon dioxide tension. 2·5% carbon dioxide in oxygen is usually satisfactory during normothermic perfusions, but a higher concentration of carbon dioxide is required when the body temperature is reduced and the metabolic rate falls (pp. 133 and 168). These gas mixtures can produce arterial oxygen tensions of 25–40 kPa (several hundred mm Hg) depending on the equipment, the flow rate and the tissue oxygen consumption. Arterial oxygen tensions of this magnitude accentuate peripheral vasoconstriction and predispose to the formation of bubbles, but they also increase the volume of oxygen carried in solution. This can be important when the haematocrit is low, and a high arterial oxygen tension is generally considered acceptable.

Some alkali is required in the priming fluid to preserve a physiological pH. Although the pH can be checked if necessary before perfusion starts, measurements of gas tensions in a blood-free prime are virtually meaningless, and assessment of blood gas and acid–base status is often delayed until blood has mixed with the electrolyte solution at the beginning of perfusion.

Recirculation and the elimination of air bubbles

The entire extracorporeal circuit must be filled with priming solution before it can be connected to the patient. This eliminates air bubbles and allows the apparatus to be checked for leaks. The prime is circulated through the sash at a flow rate which is comparable with that which will be used during perfusion, while equipment such as the heat exchanger and filters are agitated to dislodge bubbles adherent to their walls. The prime can be heated very gently if hypothermia is not required during operation, but if it is heated too much gas bubbles can be driven out of solution. This hazard is minimised if gas is not supplied to the oxygenator during recirculation, but most membrane oxygenators require a continuous flow of gas through them to prevent water condensing in the gas circuit. Gas is also supplied to *all* oxygenators during recirculation when blood has been included in the priming volume.

Connection of the extracorporeal system to the patient

Once the circuit has been primed and air has been eliminated, the pump is stopped. The sash tubing can then be clamped by the surgeon and divided.

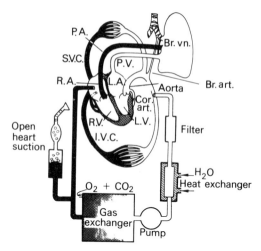

Figure 8.6 Schematic diagram representing the extracorporeal circuit and its connection to the patient, reproduced by courtesy of Mr P. E. Ghadiali.

The arterial end is joined to the aortic or femoral cannula, taking particular care to eliminate air bubbles. Blood cannot flow back into the oxygenator because it is obstructed by the pump rollers, but pressure transients should be transmitted freely to the manometer on the arterial line. The venous cannulae are joined to a Y-piece and the stem of this is attached to the other end of the cut sash tubing. Air bubbles in this tubing should also be avoided as far as possible because they can obstruct blood flow when perfusion starts, and may be carried through into the arterial blood, particularly if a membrane oxygenator is being used. The venous line enters the oxygenator through a choke which can totally occlude the tubing when necessary. This must remain clamped until bypass is commenced, otherwise the patient will be exsanguinated into the oxygenator.

Perfusion is started when all the connections have been completed satisfactorily and a check has been made to ensure that none of the lines are clamped. The choke on the venous return is gradually opened, and at the same time the flow rate from the arterial pump is increased so that the level of blood in the oxygenator does not alter and the venous pressures remain unchanged. Mixing the patient's blood with the priming solution occurs at this stage and should be carried out slowly. If the heart is still ejecting, blood from the left ventricle will preferentially reach the cerebral vessels and maintain a flow of fully oxygenated blood to the brain rather than perfusing it with pure electrolyte solution directly out of the oxygenator.

The arterial pressure is often barely altered for as long as some blood passes through the heart and is ejected into the aorta. Once left ventricular ejection ceases, the mean pressure generally falls and quite severe hypotension

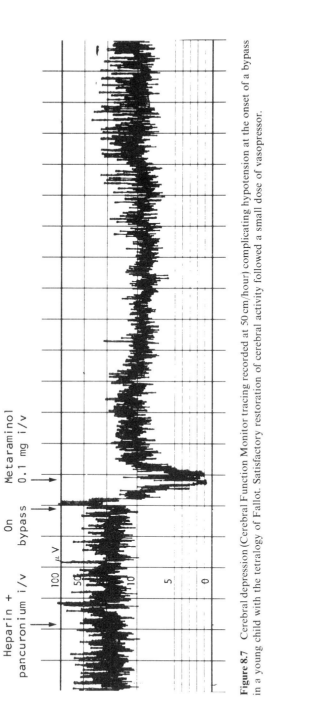

Figure 8.7 Cerebral depression (Cerebral Function Monitor tracing recorded at 50 cm/hour) complicating hypotension at the onset of a bypass in a young child with the tetralogy of Fallot. Satisfactory restoration of cerebral activity followed a small dose of vasopressor.

e.g. 25–40 mm Hg, (3·3–5.3 kPa) can occur, even though the systemic flow rate is high. This fall in pressure is particularly noticeable if the heart fails abruptly. It is due in part to the reduction in viscosity caused by haemodilution and to the dilution of circulating catecholamines; it is accentuated if there is aortic regurgitation which permits blood to run back into the left ventricle, or if there is an aortopulmonary communication such as an unrecognised patent ductus arteriosus or widely patent bronchopulmonary collateral vessels. Many patients can tolerate quite profound falls in systemic blood pressure but others can not. Sudden blanching of the face, dilatation of the pupils or a change in the level of cerebral activity as monitored on an EEG or Cerebral Function Monitor are indications for raising the pressure. Increasing the flow from the oxygenator is rarely effective, even if it is possible, and a small dose of a vasopressor, e.g. metaraminol 1 mg, is often necessary.

REGULATION OF FLOW RATE AND VASCULAR TONE DURING EXTRACORPOREAL CIRCULATION

The systemic flow supplied during cardiopulmonary bypass should be sufficient to meet tissue oxygen requirements and prevent the generation of a metabolic acidosis. It is difficult to define an optimum value because oxygen consumption is influenced by anaesthesia and often by hypothermia, arterial oxygen content is decreased by haemodilution, and tissue perfusion depends on the systemic pressure and the distribution of blood within the vascular bed as well as on the total flow rate.

In practice, a metabolic acidosis is likely to develop during normothermic perfusion if the flow rate is less than $2·4 \, \mathrm{l} \, \mathrm{m}^{-2} \mathrm{min}^{-1}$. Higher flows are often used, calculated on the basis of body weight (e.g. $80 \, \mathrm{ml} \, \mathrm{kg}^{-1} \mathrm{min}^{-1}$), but ultimately flow is limited by either the size of the arterial cannula or by the design of the oxygenator. Oxygen uptake is incomplete if blood transit time through the machine is too fast, and with disc and bubble oxygenators, high flow rates are likely to sweep air bubbles into the arterial line.

High flow rates do not ensure good tissue perfusion. The systemic vascular resistance often falls abruptly at the onset of bypass, but thereafter it tends to rise, possibly because of high arterial oxygen tensions, or as a response to the non-pulsatile waveform, or because there is a rising level of circulating catecholamines during the procedure. This tendency to vasoconstriction is augmented by hypothermia, and if it is unchecked, the arterial blood pressure rises, the volume of blood in the extracorporeal apparatus increases and tissue perfusion deteriorates as evidenced by the development of a metabolic acidosis and a falling urinary output. Anaesthetic drugs with vasodilating properties are often chosen to offset this tendency (e.g. morphine, droperidol).

Alternatively, chlorpromazine (2·5–10 mg) or phentolamine (1–2 mg) can be added to the blood in the oxygenator.

DRUG THERAPY DURING PERFUSION

A number of drugs may be needed during perfusion. The majority have been discussed in preceding sections, but all are summarised here for convenience.

Anaesthetic agents (p. 88) Small incremental doses of narcotic analgesics and muscle relaxants are given at the onset of bypass; inhalational anaesthetics are sometimes added to the gas supplied to the oxygenator.

Anticoagulants A constant level of heparinisation must be maintained, and unless facilities are available for rapidly and accurately estimating heparin activity (p. 84), additional doses of heparin (1 mg/kg) are given every hour. ACD or CPD blood added during perfusion is heparinised and calcium levels are reconstituted before use (p. 144).

Fluids, electrolytes and diuretics Some renal damage may occur during cardiopulmonary bypass, but significant impairment of renal function is unlikely if a high urinary output is maintained throughout. A diuresis may be established spontaneously if there is considerable haemodilution and good tissue perfusion, but diuretics are often given too, either manitol 25 ml of a 20% solution every hour or a single dose of frusemide 40–80 mg at the onset of bypass.

Electrolyte solutions or 5% dextrose are added to replace the urine passed and so keep the haematocrit low during perfusion.

Potassium loss is replaced in a dose which depends on urinary output and serial measurements of the plasma potassium concentration. Potassium requirements decrease if a metabolic acidosis develops. Sodium bicarbonate should be given if a metabolic acidosis of more than 5 mmol/l is detected, and at the same time the cause for the acidosis should be sought and corrected if possible.

Vasoactive drugs A short-acting vasopressor is sometimes needed immediately after the onset of bypass if the cerebral circulation appears to be jeopardised by hypotension (p. 148). Thereafter, the systemic vascular resistance is likely to increase and vasodilating agents may be required to ensure good tissue perfusion (p. 148–9). Towards the end of bypass, drug therapy may be needed to control dysrhythmias or to improve myocardial function. These are discussed on pp. 92 and 94.

Corticosteroids   It is claimed that corticosteroids in large doses (e.g. methyl prednisolone 30 mg/kg) stabilise cell and lysosomal membranes and may therefore alleviate tissue damage inflicted by ischaemia or by enzymes liberated from white cell aggregates. Large doses of methyl prednisolone are sometimes given prophylactically, particularly to high risk patients with severe pulmonary or pulmonary vascular disease, or to patients in whom some circulatory crisis complicates the operation.

HYPOTHERMIA

The historical role of hypothermia has been noted earlier in this chapter and the technique of surface cooling as a prelude to open heart surgery in infancy is described in detail in Chapter 9. Hypothermia is also used in combination with cardiopulmonary bypass. It is customary to classify the temperature reduction as mild (down to 28°C), moderate (to 20°C), or profound (below 20°C), although these figures are arbitrary and have no particular physiological significance.

Mild hypothermia is used to reduce systemic oxygen requirements so that full saturation of arterial blood can be achieved more easily, and ischaemic damage is less likely to occur if the circulation is interrupted inadvertently.

Moderate hypothermia is used to protect the myocardium during periods of ischaemic arrest and to permit perfusion at low flow rates during cardiac surgery in infancy. If only the myocardium is at risk, the whole body can be cooled or the heart can be excluded from the circulation by aortic cross-clamping, and then cooled by flooding the pericardial and cardiac cavities with iced Ringer lactate solution. The temperature of the myocardium falls more rapidly if blood stream cooling is used initially. This can then be followed by local cooling with iced Ringer lactate solution while the rest of the body is rewarmed.

Profound hypothermia is reserved for operations in which total circulatory arrest is necessary, for example surgery on the ascending aorta or aortic arch, or intricate procedures carried out in infancy when the presence of the cannulae prevents satisfactory access. Perfusion is discontinued when the core temperature reaches 15–20°C and surgery is completed on a motionless heart. During the arrest, the pupils are widely dilated and the EEG is flat in adult patients (cf. infancy, p. 168). Rewarming is started when the circulation is re-established after a period of circulatory arrest which should not exceed 1 hour at 15°C. An alternative technique for inducing profound hypothermia was popularised by Drew. It was developed when the gas transfer capacity of extracorporeal oxygenators was limited, and requires the use of separate pumps to replace the function of the left and right ventricles, while the patient's lungs continue to oxygenate the blood. Body temperature is reduced by cooling blood which is drained from the left atrium and then returned to the systemic circulation. When the heart fails, a second pump is used to deliver the systemic venous blood to the pulmonary artery. Cooling continues until the circulation is arrested at 15°C or lower. The technique is rarely used now because the time available for surgery is limited and there is a high incidence of postoperative pulmonary dysfunction, possibly related to high pressures generated in the pulmonary circuit, to embolic damage in the lungs, or to the direct effects of cold.

Mild hypothermia is generally considered to increase the safety of perfusion, but profound hypothermia carries a number of disadvantages. Although systemic oxygen requirements are decreased, the oxygen supply may fall to a greater extent because cooling induces vasoconstriction and also causes a shift to the left in the haemoglobin dissociation curve. Temperature gradients can be created between well perfused and poorly perfused tissues unless the fall in temperature is gradual, and the poorly perfused, inadequately cooled tissues contribute to the development of a metabolic acidosis during recovery. The duration of bypass is prolonged by the time taken for cooling and rewarming and there appears to be a high incidence of coagulation disturbances after perfusion at very low temperatures. Finally, there is some evidence that profound hypothermia and circulatory arrest can cause cerebral damage, particularly if the temperature of the brain is reduced by rapid blood stream cooling. The duration and intensity of action of some anaesthetic agents are influenced by hypothermia but this is rarely of practical importance; hyperglycaemia is a notable feature if large volumes of 5% dextrose solution have been given because glucose metabolism is impaired at low body temperatures.

Hypothermia is induced during bypass by regulating the temperature of the water circulating through the heat exchanger. If only a small reduction in body temperature is required, the prime in the extracorporeal circuit is allowed to remain at room temperature and the body temperature gradually drifts down as the prime mixes with the blood volume. Active cooling is necessary if the temperature is to be decreased below 30°C, and is monitored by siting temperature probes on the heat exchanger and the arterial return, as well as in the patient. Good tissue perfusion is ensured by the liberal use of vasodilating drugs and by preserving a normal arterial carbon dioxide tension. Allowance must be made for the discrepancy between the carbon dioxide tension measured in a cuvette at 37°C and the corresponding tension in a hypothermic patient (Fig. 8.8).

Rewarming is started when the intracardiac surgery has been completed and while the heart is being closed. Vasodilator drugs are continued to ensure uniform tissue perfusion and to prevent the central temperature rising rapidly while the peripheral tissues remain cold and vasoconstricted. A metabolic acidosis is often detected at this stage, but the magnitude of the base deficit

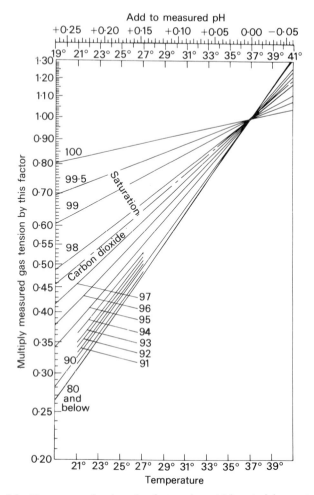

Figure 8.8 Nomogram showing the factors by which arterial gas tensions measured at 37°C must be multiplied to correct for the effect of temperature. The factors for oxygen tension depend on the saturation of haemoglobin. From Kelman & Nunn, 1966. Reproduced by permission of the Editor, *Journal of Applied Physiology.*

decreases subsequently if good tissue perfusion can be maintained. Sodium bicarbonate may be required in some cases, particularly if myocardial function is poor.

If perfusion is discontinued while the peripheral tissues are still cold, the central temperature tends to fall again in the postperfusion period. Vasodilatation continues gradually and the blood pressure falls unless transfusion is continued in excess of the measured loss. A sudden drop in pressure is particularly likely to follow the administration of protamine because of its vasodilating properties. Later in the postperfusion period, the phenomenon of 'heparin rebound' may be apparent because heparinised blood is returned from previously vasoconstricted tissues (p. 185).

For these reasons, it is desirable to warm the patient as fully as possible before bypass is discontinued. Thereafter, efforts are made to keep the body temperature normal. Stored blood is warmed before transfusion, unnecessary exposure is avoided and the patient should be transferred to a warmed bed at the end of the operation. The final stages of rewarming are often only completed in the early postoperative period.

REFERENCES

GENERAL PRINCIPLES

CLEMENT A. J. (1971) The physiological background of an apparatus used for extracorporeal circulation. *British Journal of Anaesthesia* **43**, 233.

IONESCU M. & WOOLER G. H. (1975) *Current Techniques in Extracorporeal Circulation.* Butterworths, London.

REED C. C. & CLARK D. K. (1975) *Cardiopulmonary Perfusion.* Texas Medical Press, Houston.

SELECTION AND MAINTENANCE OF EQUIPMENT

BETHUNE D. W., GILL R. D. & WHEELDON D. R. (1975) Performance of heat exchangers used in whole body perfusion circuits. *Thorax* **30**, 569.

DUNN J., KIRSH M. M., HARNESS J., CARROLL M., STRAKER J. & SLOAN H. (1974) Hemodynamic, metabolic, and hematologic effects of pulsatile cardiopulmonary bypass. *Journal of Thoracic and Cardiovascular Surgery* **68**, 138.

FREEMAN R. & KING B. (1975) Analysis of results of catheter tip cultures in open heart surgery patients. *Thorax* **30**, 26.

GELDOF W. Ch. P. & BROM A. G. (1972) Infections through blood from heart-lung machine. *Thorax* **27**, 395.

WRIGHT J. S., FISK G. C., TORDA T. A., STACEY R. B. & NICKS R. G. (1975) Some advantages of the membrane oxygenator for open heart surgery. *Journal of Thoracic and Cardiovascular Surgery* **69**, 884.

METABOLIC REQUIREMENTS AND THE REGULATION OF FLOW RATE AND VASCULAR TONE

BAILEY D. R., MILLER E. D. Jr., KAPLAN J. A. & ROGERS P. W. (1975) The renin angiotensin aldosterone system during cardiac surgery with morphine nitrous oxide anesthesia. *Anesthesiology* **42**, 538.

GORDON R. J., RAVIN M., RAWITSCHER R. E. & DAICOFF G. R. (1975) Changes in arterial pressure, viscosity, and resistance during cardiopulmonary bypass. *Journal of Thoracic and Cardiovascular Surgery* **69**, 552.

HARRIS E. A., SEELYE E. R. & BARRATT-BOYES B. G. (1970) Respiratory and metabolic acid-base changes during cardiopulmonary bypass. *British Journal of Anaesthesia* **42**, 912.

HARRIS E. A., SEELYE E. R. & SQUIRE A. W. (1971) Oxygen consumption during cardiopulmonary bypass with moderate hypothermia in man. *British Journal of Anaesthesia* **43**, 1113.

HARRIS E. A., SEELYE E. R. & BARRATT-BOYES B. G. (1974) On the availability of oxygen to the body during cardiopulmonary bypass in man. *British Journal of Anaesthesia* **46**, 425.

HINE I. P., WOOD W. G., MAINWARING-BURTON R. W., BUTLER M. J., IRVING M. H. & BOOKER B. (1976) The adrenergic response to surgery involving cardiopulmonary bypass, as measured by plasma and urinary catecholamine concentrations. *British Journal of Anaesthesia* **48**, 355.

MUIR A. L. & DAVIDSON I. A. (1971) Hypoxaemia during cardiopulmonary bypass. *Thorax* **26**, 443.

PATTERSON R. W. (1976) Effect of P_aCO_2 on oxygen consumption during cardiopulmonary bypass in man. *Current Researches in Anesthesia and Analgesia* **55**, 269.

TAN C. K., GLISSON S. N., EL-ETR A. A. & RAMANKRISHNAIAH K. B. (1976) Levels of circulating norepinephrine and epinephrine before, during, and after cardiopulmonary bypass in man. *Journal of Thoracic and Cardiovascular Surgery* **71**, 928.

CORONARY PERFUSION AND TECHNIQUES OF MYOCARDIAL PRESERVATION

BALIBREA J. L., BULLON A., DE LA FUENTE A., DE LA F. ALARCON A., FARINAS J., COLLANTES P., GIL M., GOMBAU M., MORALES R. & SANCHEZ F. (1975) Myocardial ultrastructural changes during extracorporeal circulation with anoxic cardiac arrest and its prevention by coronary perfusion. *Thorax* **30**, 371.

BUSUTTIL R. W., GEORGE W. J. & HEWITT R. L. (1975) Protective effect of methylprednisolone on the heart during ischemic arrest. *Journal of Thoracic and Cardiovascular Surgery* **70**, 955.

HEDLEY-BROWN A., BRAIMBRIDGE M. V., DARRACOTT S., CHAYEN J. & KASSAP H. (1974) An experimental evaluation of continuous normothermic, intermittent hypothermic and intermittent normothermic coronary perfusion. *Thorax* **29**, 38.

MALONEY J. V. Jr. & NELSON R. L. (1975) Myocardial preservation during cardiopulmonary bypass: an overview. *Journal of Thoracic and Cardiovascular Surgery* **70**, 1040.

HYPOTHERMIA

FELDMAN S. A. (1971) Profound hypothermia. *British Journal of Anaesthesia* **43**, 244.

HOWAT D. D. C., BARKER J., VALE R. J. & ELLIS F. R. (1973) Temperature regulation: a symposium on the use of induced hypothermia, the importance of normothermia in the surgical period, and malignant hyperthermia. *Anaesthesia* **28**, 236.

KELMAN G. R. & NUNN J. F. (1966) Nomograms for correction of blood PO_2, PCO_2, pH and base excess for time and temperature. *Journal of Applied Physiology* **21**, 1484.

MACDONALD D. J. F. (1975) Current practice of hypothermia in British cardiac surgery. *British Journal of Anaesthesia* **47**, 1011.

CHAPTER 9

ANAESTHESIA FOR CARDIAC SURGERY IN THE FIRST YEAR OF LIFE

Congenital heart disease, with an estimated incidence of 6–8/1000 live births, is a major cause of mortality in the first year of life (infancy). Without treatment, about 50% of these children die before their first birthday, one-third of the deaths occurring in the first 3 months of life.

Palliative procedures can improve the prognosis of some lesions, but even with good palliative surgery the combined risks of palliation and subsequent corrective surgery are often very high. With recent advances in open heart surgery, it is becoming increasingly common to attempt total correction as the primary procedure at an early age. This is reflected in the increasing number of infants operated on in recent years with the aid of cardiopulmonary bypass (Fig. 9.1).

There are a number of features which distinguish cardiac surgery in infancy from operations carried out in adult patients. Many of the congenital

lesions are complex and some are associated with gross haemodynamic disturbances. However, the myocardium itself is initially healthy in the vast
majority of cases, and the prognosis is correspondingly good provided the
haemodynamic lesions can be corrected and secondary changes (particularly
in the pulmonary vasculature) have not progressed too far. Arterial hypoxaemia is a feature of congenital heart disease with a right to left shunt, but
compensatory mechanisms develop over the course of time (p. 18) and

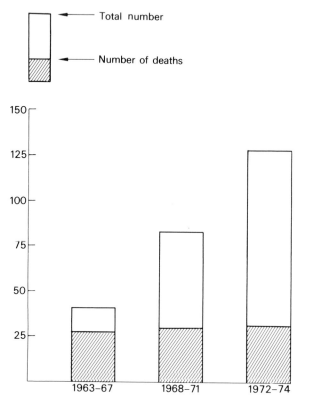

Figure 9.1   Open heart surgery in the first year of life at the Hospital for Sick
Children, Great Ormond Street, 1963–74. From Stark, 1976.

hypoxia from this cause is less hazardous than the same degree of arterial
desaturation related to pulmonary disorders. Finally, cardiac surgery in infancy entails all the problems associated with this age group—technical difficulties because of size, relative immaturity of the kidneys, a blood volume
and daily fluid turnover which are a high proportion of total body fluids, and
poorly developed homeostatic mechanisms, manifest most commonly as
hypothermia or hypoglycaemia.

DIAGNOSTIC PROCEDURES

Surgery for congenital heart disease can only be undertaken safely if the precise abnormalities have been defined by cardiac catheterisation and angiocardiography. Delay in diagnosis or treatment may prove fatal, and no infant should be considered too small or too ill for investigation. For the same reason, facilities for both catheterisation and surgery must be available at any time.

Lesions which are particularly likely to cause severe functional disturbance at an early age include transposition of the great arteries, coarctation of the aorta, pulmonary atresia, aortic stenosis, aorto-pulmonary window and total anomalous pulmonary venous drainage. These infants commonly present with severe congestive cardiac failure, pulmonary oedema or gross hypoxaemia and acidosis, often within the first month of life (neonatal period). Immediate assessment should include body temperature, blood sugar, calcium and electrolyte levels, haematocrit and the investigation of blood gas and acid–base disturbances. Blood should be sent at once for cross-matching. Hypoglycaemia and hypocalcaemia commonly warrant treatment. If the blood sugar is less than 2 mmol/l in a full term newborn neonate, or less than 1·5 mmol/l in a premature neonate, 50% dextrose should be given intravenously in a dose of 0·2 ml/kg. If the serum calcium concentration is less than 1·5 mmol/l, intravenous calcium gluconate should be given (0·225 mmol). Oxygen in high concentration should be administered initially to all severely ill babies with suspected congenital heart disease and is safe for the relatively short time which elapses before investigation and surgery. However, if cyanosis is caused by a large right to left intracardiac shunt, oxygen therapy will only have a relatively slight effect on the arterial oxygen tension. Very sick infants occasionally require endotracheal intubation and intermittent positive pressure ventilation (IPPV) prior to investigation.

Cardiac catheterisation and angiocardiography in infancy are usually carried out without general anaesthesia. The catheter is passed into the saphenous vein, the saphenofemoral function, or occasionally into the axillary vein, after local infiltration with 1% lignocaine. Sedation is often unnecessary in the newborn neonate; alternatively, chloral hydrate (75 mg/kg) can be given via a nasogastric tube. Supplements of diazepam (0·1 mg/kg) can be given intravenously via the cardiac catheter if necessary.

Heavier sedation is usually required beyond the immediate newborn period. In the first month of life, Pethidine Co. (0·05 ml/kg) can be given intramuscularly 30 minutes before catheterisation. Each ml contains pethidine 25 mg, promethazine 6·25 mg and chlorpromazine 6·25 mg. In older infants, the dose can be increased to 0·1 ml/kg. It is helpful to give children over 6 months of age an oral sedative such as phenobarbitone (2 mg/kg) the night before investigation, and either to repeat this or use trimeprazine (Vallergan)

3–4 mg/kg orally 4 hours prior to catheterisation. Intramuscular premedication is then given as described above. This technique generally provides optimal sedation and analgesia without respiratory or cardiovascular depression. The infant continues to breathe air, so facilitating the interpretation of differences in oxygen saturation in blood drawn from various sites within the circulation (p. 42).

General anaesthesia is seldom required, but if it is considered essential, endotracheal intubation, muscle relaxants and IPPV should be used; it is preferable to avoid increasing the inspired oxygen concentration beyond 33%.

The hazards of cardiac catheterisation in infancy include hypothermia, haemorrhage, allergic reactions to contrast materials, trauma to the heart or great vessels, and dysrhythmias. Newborn infants, particularly those born prematurely, are especially susceptible to heat loss in a cold environment and are poorly equipped to deal with it. The temperature of the room in which catheterisation is performed should be not less than 24°C. The infant should be swathed in warm clothing and, if possible, should lie on a radiolucent warming pad. In babies particularly at risk, the limbs should also be wrapped in silver foil which helps to retain heat.

The blood volume in infancy is approximately 85 ml/kg and loss of more than 10% of the total generally requires replacement. In small infants, excessive amounts can easily be removed during blood sampling unless oximetry is carried out in a sterilised cuvette from which the sample can be returned to the child.

'Allergic reactions' including hypotension are rare after the injection of modern angiographic contrast media and the total dose can be as high as 4–5 ml/kg. Hypotension is more commonly related to blood loss, or to dysrhythmias occurring as a result of intracardiac manipulations of the catheter. If there is a right to left shunt, flow through it may increase if the systemic pressure falls, and central cyanosis will become more intense. Alternatively, cyanosis can be accentuated because the tone of the outflow tract of the right ventricle increases ('infundibular spasm') so causing a greater proportion of blood to be deflected through a patent interventricular septum. This causes, rather than is caused by, systemic hypotension. Infundibular spasm can be relieved by sedation with opiates (morphine sulphate 0·2 mg/kg) or by β-adrenergic blocking drugs such as propranolol in 0·01 mg/kg increments to a maximum dose of 0·1 mg/kg. Extreme hypotension should be treated with pressor agents.

Occasionally, one of the great vessels or even the heart itself is punctured by the catheter; this may result in life-threatening haemorrhage but sometimes is only recognised when blood-stained fluid is found in the pericardial cavity at the time of surgery.

The mortality which can be attributed directly to cardiac catheterisation and angiocardiography in infancy has now been reduced to less than 1%. When investigation is required in the first month of life, the in-hospital mortality is considerably greater than 1%, but the hazards of catheterisation cannot be separated clearly from those of either the cardiac lesion or its treatment.

The usual resuscitative measures are required if cardiac arrest does occur during catheterisation; particular care should be taken to avoid excessive heat loss, and to correct metabolic acidosis in infants with gross arterial desaturation.

OPERATIVE PROCEDURES

Premedication

Infants with congenital heart disease generally tolerate premedication well and careful preoperative sedation will allow the use of reduced doses of general anaesthetic agents. Intramuscular Pethidine Co. 0·07 ml/kg with atropine according to weight (Table 9.1), or papaveretum 0·3–0·4 mg/kg and hyoscine 0·006–0·008 mg/kg are both satisfactory combinations.

Table 9.1   Atropine dosage in infancy

Weight (kg)	Dose (μg)
Up to 2·5	150
2·5–8·0	200
8·0–15·0	300
15·0–20·0	400

Induction of anaesthesia

There are a number of techniques available for the induction of anaesthesia in infancy, and the choice is often determined by the clinical condition of the baby. The sickest infants, especially those in the neonatal period, may require endotracheal intubation and artificial ventilation before they reach the operating theatre. Stronger neonates, particularly in the first week of life, may be intubated without difficulty while they are awake. If they are vigorous, it may be wiser to intubate using muscle relaxants, with or without light general anaesthesia. Outside the neonatal period, induction of light general anaesthesia and intubation with the aid of muscle relaxants are usually required. If the superficial veins are prominent as they often are in thin children with congenital heart disease, intravenous thiopentone (4–6 mg/kg) can be given, followed by either suxamethonium (1 mg/kg) or pancuronium bromide

(0·1–0·2 mg/kg). An inhalational induction is favoured in many experienced paediatric centres. A well sedated infant can generally be anaesthetised with 50% nitrous oxide in oxygen, but cyclopropane in oxygen is widely regarded as the technique of choice. Although the mixture is explosive and cannot be continued for long, induction is smooth and rapid with minimal disturbance of the blood pressure. Cyclopropane is particularly valuable for patients with the tetralogy of Fallot because it alleviates infundibular spasm. Halothane is less satisfactory and is contraindicated in infants with any form of left ventricular outflow tract obstruction because hypotension and ventricular fibrillation occur very readily. Hypotension is particularly dangerous during induction because monitoring is much less intense.

Table 9.2   Approximate dimensions of oral endotracheal tubes used in infancy

Age	Internal diameter (mm)	Length (cm)
Premature newborn	2·5	8–9
Full-term newborn	3·0	8–9
1–3 months	3·0–3·5	9–10
3–12 months	3·5–4·0	10–11
1–2 years	4·0–4·5	11–12

It is unwise to deepen inhalational anaesthesia to the point where intubation can be carried out without coughing. Instead, suxamethonium or pancuronium are given intravenously in the doses quoted above, or intramuscular suxamethonium (2 mg/kg) can be used if the superficial veins are difficult to identify. Non-cuffed endotracheal tubes are used to minimise tracheal damage. The size is selected according to age rather than weight (Table 9.2) because many of these infants are very small for their age, but the larynx has developed fairly normally. Either oral or nasal tubes can be chosen. The advantage of the former is that they can be introduced more easily and hypoxia is less likely to occur, but a nasal tube can be secured in place with greater safety for postoperative care. The ideal arrangement is to intubate initially with an oral tube and then change to a plastic nasal tube later if IPPV is to be continued postoperatively (p. 171). Endotracheal tubes can be dislodged or disconnected with particular ease in infants and small children, and it is important to check that the tube is the correct length for the child and that the endotracheal connector cannot be removed easily. Methods for securing oral and nasal tubes are illustrated in Figs. 9.2 and 9.3.

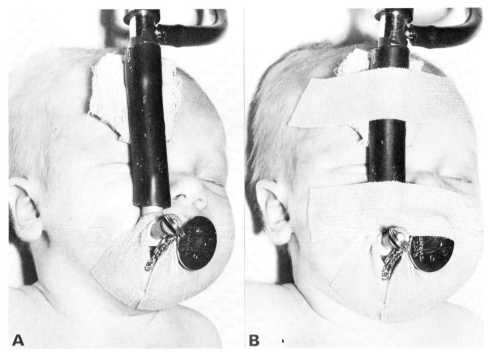

Figure 9.2 Fixation of orotracheal tube, stages A and B.

Maintenance of anaesthesia

Intermittent positive pressure ventilation is continued using 50% nitrous oxide in oxygen as the basic anaesthetic mixture. Non-depolarising relaxants are given to facilitate the control of ventilation, smaller doses being required if depolarising agents have been used for intubation (e.g. pancuronium 0·06–0·08 mg/kg or *d*-tubocurarine 0·4 mg/kg). Narcotic supplements are sometimes necessary, e.g. pethidine 0·5–1·0 mg/kg, morphine 0·1–0·2 mg/kg, or halothane up to 0·5%; the latter should be used with caution because of the risks of hypotension and myocardial depression.

The number of mechanical ventilators which are suitable for infants has increased considerably in the last few years. The requirements for operating theatre use include a simple mechanism for changing from IPPV to manual ventilation and an easily accessible, high-flow oxygen bypass. Good humidification is essential and the macine should be reliable and quiet. When the infant is connected to the ventilator, the respiratory frequency is usually set between 24 and 30 breaths per minute and the tidal volume should be adjusted so that adequate chest movement is visible, rather than by reference to complex nomograms.

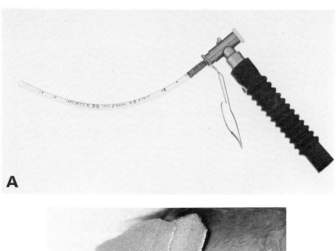

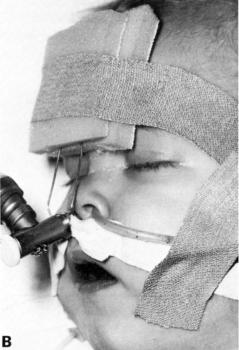

Figure 9.3 A, Nasotracheal tube with Tunstall connector and Oxford swivel; B, Fixation of a nasotracheal tube.

Monitoring

The monitoring described for closed cardiac surgery in adult patients is less sophisticated than that used during open heart surgery. In general, the same distinction does not apply in infancy because the procedures are often associated with considerable risk and the patient's condition is serious before surgery is commenced.

The ECG is monitored throughout all operations and a reliable intravenous infusion is essential. This should be established as soon as possible after the induction of anaesthesia so that anaesthetic agents or resuscitative drugs can be given easily if required. Siting the venous cannula in a central vein (femoral, internal or external jugular) permits monitoring of the central venous pressure. This may not be essential during surgery but is a great help if the infant's condition is unsatisfactory in the postoperative period. Not only can the venous pressure be monitored but cannulae in central veins are dislodged less easily than those in peripheral vessels. It is much easier to set up the infusion while the infant is anaesthetised and therefore generally desirable to cannulate a central vein from the outset. Catheters inserted *percutaneously* in the antecubital fossa can rarely be advanced to the superior vena cava in infants, and both the failure rate and the morbidity associated with direct cannulation of the central veins are greater than in adults. If the jugular or femoral vessels cannot be cannulated easily, it is wiser to *cut-down* on a vein in a limb and advance a catheter into one or other cava. Measurement of the superior vena caval pressure is essential during cardiopulmonary bypass, and it may be necessary to monitor pressure in both jugular veins if there is a persistent left superior vena cava. This is because cannulation of the left superior vena cava will be required during bypass if clamping the vessel leads to a rise in pressure in the left internal jugular vein. Cannulation of any vein draining to the superior vena cava is contraindicated in patients requiring a Glenn procedure for the palliation of tricuspid atresia (p. 124).

Continuous monitoring of the arterial blood pressure is essential during open heart surgery and is desirable during closed cardiac procedures on sick neonates. Percutaneous arterial cannulation is possible in many infants, even neonates, provided a fine cannula is used (e.g. 22 F). This is generally inserted into the radial or brachial artery, although the ulnar artery can be used in older children. Major complications of arterial cannulation at the wrist are rare, possibly because the arterial wall is healthier in children, or because there is a better collateral blood supply. However, cannulation should not be attempted if there are deformities of the wrist or hand, or if the radial and ulnar arteries cannot be palpated easily.

It is desirable to monitor core temperature during all surgery in infants, and a temperature probe can be placed in either the pharynx or the rectum. During open heart surgery and elective hypothermia, the temperature of the blood and the myocardium is estimated with a probe situated in the mid-oesophagus, close to the left atrium.

An oesophageal stethoscope is helpful sometimes, especially if the ECG is not supplemented with intra-arterial pressure monitoring. It also permits auscultation of the breath sounds.

A urinary catheter is inserted before open heart surgery, but urine can be collected in an adhesive bag during shorter operations. Monitoring the electroencephalograph with the Cerebral Function Monitor (p. 86) is a useful adjunct for the control of either low flow cardiopulmonary bypass, or circulatory arrest during profound hypothermia (p. 168).

CLOSED CARDIAC SURGERY

Many of the closed cardiac procedures carried out in infancy are palliative operations which are discussed in the sections devoted to the appropriate specific condition. Two definitive procedures which may be required at this age are closure of a patent ductus arteriosus and resection of coarctation of the aorta. The management of these conditions in adult patients is discussed in Chapter 5, but the problems presented in infancy differ considerably and are described below.

Closure of patent ductus arteriosus

In 20–25% of cases, a patent ductus arteriosus is large enough to cause a substantial left to right shunt and gives rise to symptoms in infancy. Repeated chest infections occur and cardiac enlargement and heart failure are common. Many of these infants require antibiotics, digitalis and diuretics preoperatively and there is a significant mortality in spite of medical treatment.

When the child is ready for surgery, the ductus is closed through a left thoracotomy. The anaesthetic technique should be as for any sick infant with controlled ventilation and light anaesthesia throughout. Postoperative respiratory complications are common, and a prolonged period of endotracheal intubation and mechanical ventilation may be required.

The ductus commonly remains patent in association with other congenital cardiac anomalies such as transposition of the great arteries, coarctation of the aorta, atrial or ventricular septal defect or pulmonary stenosis. It is essential for the nature of these associated lesions to be defined before the duct is ligated. A significant proportion of the pulmonary blood flow may be derived through the ductus if this remains patent in infants with transposition of the great arteries, and in preductal coarctation the ductus may be carrying much of the blood supply to the lower part of the body. If an attempt is made to establish cardiopulmonary bypass in the presence of an undiagnosed patent ductus, flow through the low resistance pathway of the ductus and lungs increases enormously, rapidly distending the left heart and preventing maintenance of a normal systemic pressure. This situation can occasionally be difficult to control if the ductus is relatively inaccessible through a medium sternotomy. Closure of the ductus may therefore be required as a prelude to further surgery.

Increasing interest has been shown recently in ligation of the ductus arteriosus in severe cases of idiopathic respiratory distress syndrome of the newborn (RDS). The ductus usually remains patent in this condition because of severe hypoxaemia, and it has been claimed that the excessive pulmonary blood flow exacerbates the disorder by decreasing pulmonary compliance. At the time of writing, the results of ligation of the ductus in infants with the respiratory distress syndrome have not been evaluated fully, but closure is generally recommended if severe RDS is complicated by cardiac failure with signs of a large flow through the ductus.

Resection of coarctation of the aorta

Coarctation in infancy is commonly preductal (p. 60). The physiological significance of this location is that the ductus arteriosus remains patent and provides much of the blood supply to the lower part of the body. Cyanosis restricted to the lower extremities is theoretically possible but most of these infants are uniformly cyanosed because the severe coarctation causes pulmonary oedema. In the worst cases, coarctation is associated with gross hypoplasia of the left ventricle or the whole of the aortic arch. Other congenital anomalies are frequently present, so increasing the threat to life of an already serious lesion. Drug therapy does little to alleviate heart failure, and surgical relief of the stenosis is the only effective form of treatment. Without operation, 75% of symptomatic infants with coarctation die in the first year of life.

The management of these sick infants creates one of the greatest challenges in paediatric anaesthesia. They often present with both cardiac and respiratory failure, suffering from hypoxaemia and even hypercapnia caused by pulmonary oedema, together with a severe metabolic acidosis. Particular care is needed during induction, and halothane should be avoided because it decreases cardiac output and increases the incidence of ventricular fibrillation; even nitrous oxide is poorly tolerated in a few cases. Manual rather than automatic ventilation is often chosen because adequate gas exchange is difficult to achieve in the presence of pulmonary oedema and an open hemithorax. Intra-arterial pressure monitoring is advisable in infants with severe heart failure, and the cannula should be introduced into the right radial or brachial artery before the induction of anaesthesia.

Resuscitative drugs and equipment should be readily accessible from the outset, although if ventricular fibrillation does occur, it is usually irreversible. Metabolic acidosis should be corrected before the aortic clamps are applied, and blood should be run through a blood warmer, ready to be given. It is wise to expand the lungs fully, ventilating with 100% oxygen for 2 to 3 minutes immediately before aortic cross-clamping. Blood can be given conveniently from a syringe using a three-way stopcock connected to the intravenous infusion set, and it is worth transfusing 10 to 20 ml in advance of any loss because even mild hypovolaemia is likely to lead to hypotension.

OPEN HEART SURGERY IN INFANCY

Cardiopulmonary bypass can now be used with relative safety, even in new-born infants, largely as a result of refinements in oxygenators, filters and in-tracardiac cannulae and suckers. Alternatively, surface cooling is induced, followed by a limited period of extracorporeal circulation leading to circula-tory arrest during profound hypothermia at a nasopharyngeal temperature of 15 to 22°C. The repair is carried out on a motionless heart and access to intracardiac structures is excellent because caval cannulae and suckers can be removed from the field during the arrest period. However, the circulation cannot be interrupted safely for more than an hour, even at 15°C, and reduc-ing core temperature to this extent may produce structural neurological damage and regional hypoxia from paralysis of autoregulatory vasomotor mechanisms.

Perfusion technique in infancy

The principles of management during perfusion do not differ significantly from those employed in adult patients which are described in detail in Chapters 6 and 8. A few points of particular importance are noted here.

Both bubble and rotating disc oxygenators can be used satisfactorily for open heart surgery in infancy although membrane oxygenators are sometimes considered preferable because of the lower incidence of damage to the blood. Fresh heparinised blood is often chosen to prime the extracorporeal circuit for surgery within the first few months of life so that the risk of coagulation disorders can be minimised, and the metabolic alkalosis which follows the transfusion of citrated blood can be avoided. Extreme haemodilution is un-desirable because of the difficulty of excreting a large fluid load, and the haematocrit is generally maintained at between 30 and 40%.

Hypothermia is often employed, generally as an adjunct to extracorporeal circulation, but sometimes before surgery begins. A common policy is to in-duce preliminary surface cooling in all infants under 3 months of age; the skin incision is made when the temperature has reached 24 to 27°C, and median sternotomy is then performed and the heart cannulated in the usual way. It is customary to cannulate both cavae in infants rather than rely on drainage through a single right atrial cannula because communication between the two sides of the heart is common in this age group even when the lesion is one in which intact septa might be expected.

The chief advantage of preliminary surface cooling is that it decreases the total time required on bypass. It also slows the heart, so making cardiac cannulation easier, while the reduction in oxygen consumption allows time for this to be completed safely, even in those comparatively rare cases in which manipulation of the heart induces ventricular fibrillation.

Technique of surface cooling in infancy

The anaesthetised infant is placed on a water blanket containing ice-cold water and ice-filled plastic bags are packed around the body. Care should be taken to avoid placing these on the precordium, or on the extremities of the limbs. Sudden movement of cold limbs should also be avoided, or alternatively, gentle massage of major muscle groups should be carried out continuously. Shivering and excessive vasoconstriction are eliminated by full muscular relaxation together with general anaesthesia, usually with nitrous oxide, oxygen and 0·25–0·5% halothane. Humidification of the respiratory tract remains essential and the temperature of the humidifier is not reduced during cooling. As the metabolic rate falls, carbon dioxide production decreases to such an extent that at constant alveolar ventilation, serious degrees of hypocapnia and respiratory alkalosis can be produced very easily. Hypokalaemia has also been reported.

It is important to note that the apparent tension of gases in the arterial blood is misleadingly high unless allowance is made for the difference in temperature between the patient and the measuring apparatus which is generally maintained at 37°C (p. 152). An arterial carbon dioxide tension of 6·7 kPa (50 mm Hg) measured at 37°C corresponds to an actual tension of 4·7 kPa (35 mm Hg) at 30°C. Hypocapnia increases the risk of cardiac dysrhythmias and therefore carbon dioxide (2·5–5%) should be added to the inspired gas mixture once the core temperature reaches 34°C; reducing the inspired minute volume rather than adding carbon dioxide predisposes to atelectasis. It is sometimes advocated that the arterial carbon dioxide tension, corrected for temperature, should be kept even higher than normal during hypothermia, for example between 6·0 and 7·3 kPa (45–55 mm Hg), to encourage cerebral vasodilatation and more rapid cerebral cooling.

Ventricular fibrillation is likely to occur if the myocardial temperature is decreased too far, and core temperature during surface cooling is therefore measured in the mid-oesophagus, behind the heart. Active cooling is discontinued once the temperature has reached 29 to 30°C; the infant is dried, drapes applied and surgery commenced. By this time, the temperature has generally drifted down to between 27 and 28°C. This after-drop is more profound if cooling has taken place rapidly, and is also more noticeable in fat infants. If surgery is carried out with the infant lying on a water blanket, fine control of body temperature can be achieved by varying the temperature of the water circulating in the blanket. However, this cannot produce rapid changes and any need for external control at this stage must be anticipated well before the temperature has drifted too far from the desired level.

Hypothermia during perfusion; profound hypothermia with circulatory arrest

Once cardiopulmonary bypass has been established, it is customary to lower body temperature still further; tissue oxygen requirements decrease to about 45% of basal at 25°C and 17% of basal at 20°C. Surgery is either carried out during complete circulatory arrest at 15–22°C, or alternatively, the temperature is maintained at 25°C while the infant is perfused at a relatively low flow rate; short periods of circulatory arrest can be tolerated without apparent harm at this temperature while particularly delicate stages of the operation are in progress.

The brain is the organ which is most at risk during periods of low flow or circulatory arrest, and once surface cooling has been completed and the risk of ventricular fibrillation has largely passed, the site of temperature monitoring is moved from the oesophagus to the nasopharynx or the external auditory meatus. These sites provide a better indication of cerebral temperature which is often higher than in the oesophagus.

If a prolonged period of circulatory arrest is planned, some indication of whether or not cerebral metabolic activity has been adequately depressed before the arrest period starts can be obtained by inspection of the Cerebral Function Monitor. The mean level of activity falls gradually from 30°C onwards until between 20 and 18°C, slow, high voltage activity appears and the mean level of the recording drops rapidly. Provided this degree of cerebral depression has been reached, cessation of cerebral perfusion does not produce an abrupt change, and cerebral electrical activity returns as soon as perfusion is recommenced (Fig. 9.4). If these precautions are not taken and circulatory arrest is permitted merely because the probe in the nasopharynx registers the desired temperature, cerebral activity is depressed abruptly at the moment of clamping and only returns slowly when perfusion starts again. There is usually electrical silence during circulatory arrest at temperatures of 15°C, although in young children burst suppression is sometimes seen throughout (Fig. 9.5).

Rewarming is started while the heart is being closed. The blood returning from the oxygenator is warmed, and at the same time warm water is circulated through the blanket on which the child is lying. This source of warmth persists after bypass has been discontinued and helps to prevent a postperfusion drop in temperature which tends to occur when cold blood returns from previously poorly perfused extremities. Care must be taken, however, to prevent damage to cold and relatively ischaemic skin; this is likely to occur if the temperature of the blanket is more than a degree or two higher than normal body temperatures. Transfusion of cold blood must also be avoided, and any blood transfused in the postperfusion period should be run through a warming coil.

Metabolic acidosis is a common concomitant of profound hypothermia, especially if combined with circulatory arrest. Serial measurements of pH and

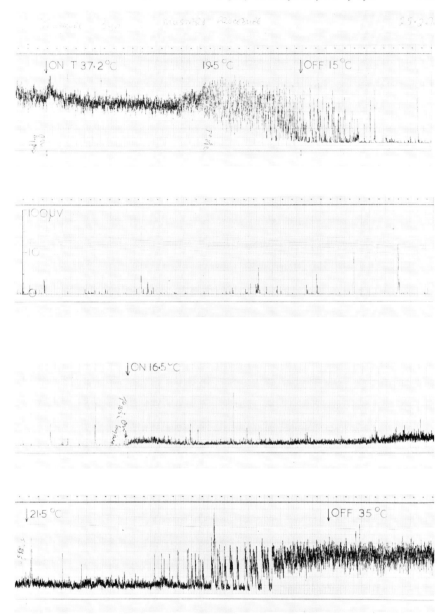

Figure 9.4   Complete record of cerebral electrical activity in a child of 3 (Cerebral Function Monitor recording at 6 mm min^{-1}) during 69 minutes of circulatory arrest at a nasopharyngeal temperature of 15°C. The record shows considerable depression of cerebral activity before the arrest and prompt recovery when the circulation is restored. A normal level has been reached before perfusion is discontinued at a temperature of 35°C.

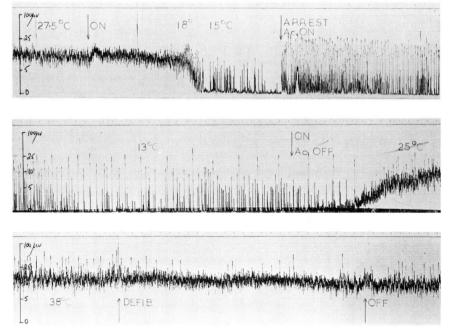

Figure 9.5 'Burst suppression' recorded on the Cerebral Function Monitor (run at 6 mm min^{-1}) throughout a 49-minute period of circulatory arrest in an 18-month-old child. Reproduced from Branthwaite, 1973, by permission of the Editor, *Anaesthesia.*

arterial blood gas tensions are required during rewarming, and correction of metabolic acidosis with sodium bicarbonate is usually necessary.

Management in the postperfusion period

An effective circulation can often be restored quite easily after cardiopulmonary bypass in infancy, provided the haemodynamic lesion has been corrected completely. Perfusion is discontinued gradually by allowing the heart to fill, while the systemic and left and right atrial pressures are observed carefully. A satisfactory output can usually be achieved when the higher of the two atrial pressures is between 10 and 15 mm Hg (1·3–2·0 kPa) relative to the mid-axillary line. 0·25 m mol of calcium (as calcium chloride) is often given as soon as perfusion is discontinued. Further myocardial support is required occasionally, either isoprenaline or adrenaline 0·5–1·0 mg in 100 ml infused from a microdrip apparatus (60 drops = 1 ml). Frusemide, 1 mg/kg, can be given intravenously if the urine output is less than 1 ml/kg/hour. Potassium supplements are required less frequently than for adult patients, possibly reflecting the lower incidence of preoperative depletion.

Anaesthesia is continued with 50% nitrous oxide in oxygen, and halothane is avoided entirely. Heparin is reversed in the usual way with protamine sulphate, and the thrombin time or blood-activated recalcification time can be estimated 20 minutes later if there is any doubt about the adequacy of coagulation mechanisms.

Postoperative management

There is a high incidence of postoperative respiratory insufficiency and hypoxaemia following open heart surgery in infancy, and all infants are ventilated via an endotracheal tube for at least a few hours and usually until the following day. If an orotracheal tube has been selected for use during the operation, it is replaced with a nasal tube at the end of operation because this is easier to secure and to manage. The tube should be made of non-irritant plastic and should be small enough to allow a slight audible leak of gas around it during intermittent positive pressure ventilation. This usually means using a tube which is 0·5 mm smaller than the one used during operation, and allows for the oedema which occurs in the subglottic region after intubation. If this step is not taken, intractable subglottic stenosis may develop in a relatively short time. Should the audible leak around the tube disappear at any time during the postoperative period, it is probably wise to change the tube for a smaller size.

The change-over from oral to nasotracheal intubation must be accomplished with the minimum disturbance to ventilation. The nasal tube is inserted through the nose into the pharynx while the orotracheal tube is still in place. Suction is applied through the nasal tube to ensure that the lumen has not become occluded during its passage through the nose, and it is then advanced under direct vision until its tip reaches the laryngeal inlet. It is cut so that a length of 3 to 4 cm protrudes from the nose and a well-fitting connector* or Bennett† is attached. After a few breaths of manual ventilation with 100% oxygen, suction is applied through the oral tube which is then withdrawn quickly. The nasal tube is advanced immediately into the trachea under direct vision. Care must be taken to avoid pressure on the alae nasae when the tube is secured, and a typical method of fixation which minimises the risk of nasal ulceration is illustrated in Fig. 9.3, p. 162. After the tube has been secured, movement and air entry on both sides of the chest are checked. It is convenient to insert a nasogastric tube through the other nostril at the same time.

During the transfer from operating theatre to intensive therapy unit, the infant is ventilated manually with oxygen; drainage tubes are clamped for the minimum possible time to avoid the risk of cardiac tamponade. On reach-

* Tunstall, Longworth Scientific Co. Ltd., Abingdon, Oxford.
† Bennett, available in the UK from Simonsen & Weel, Sidcup, Kent.

ing the ward, continuous arterial, left atrial and superior caval or right atrial pressure recordings are re-established as soon as possible, and heart rate, central and peripheral temperatures, and blood balance are charted every quarter of an hour. The urine output and osmolality are monitored, and a chest X-ray, blood and urinary electrolyte estimations are performed. The blood volume is maintained at an optimum level by transfusion; blood or plasma is given to keep the haematocrit between 30 and 40%, and inotropic drugs are used if necessary.

The infant is sedated with small intravenous, or intramuscular doses of morphine (0·2 mg/kg) or diazepam (0·2 mg/kg), and blood gas analysis is performed as soon as ventilation is stable. Positive end-expiratory pressure may be helpful if an arterial oxygen tension of 9·3 kPa (70 mm Hg) cannot be achieved with less than 60% inspired oxygen in an infant with a fully corrected haemodynamic defect. Particular attention must be paid to proper humidification and the inspired gas must be saturated with water at a temperature of approximately 35°C near the patient.

Suction is carried out regularly using a soft catheter, and normal saline (0·5 ml in infants) should be instilled through the nasal tube, every 15 minutes if necessary, to loosen tracheal secretions.

The oxygen concentration of the inspired gas is reduced when the circulation is stable, and controlled ventilation is usually discontinued 24 to 48 hours after operation. Continuous positive airway pressure (CPAP) with spontaneous respiration may be helpful in infants who remain hypoxaemic on high inspired oxygen concentrations, and during weaning from IPPV.

IMPLICATIONS OF SPECIFIC CARDIAC LESIONS IN INFANCY

Isolated pulmonary stenosis

It is occasionally necessary to relieve pulmonary stenosis in infancy. These children are frequently cyanosed because the elevated right atrial pressure prevents closure of the foramen ovale, but intractable heart failure and respiratory disorders are less common than in patients with obstruction to left ventricular ejection.

The stenosis is generally at valvar level and a satisfactory opening can usually be achieved, although it is rarely possible to leave a normally functioning valve. Some degree of pulmonary incompetence is common, but this is a haemodynamically unimportant lesion. The patent foramen ovale is closed at the same time and the results of surgery are good.

Ventricular septal defect (VSD)

Ventricular septal defects which are present in infancy often decrease in size or even close spontaneously. However, there is a significant chance of irreversible pulmonary vascular disease developing within the first 2 years of life if a large defect remains patent. The risks of corrective surgery between the ages of 1 and 2 years are now similar to those in later life, and operation should be performed before the pulmonary vascular resistance increases significantly. If necessary, this is carried out before the age of 12 months; more commonly, early surgery is required because of intractable heart failure, recurrent pneumonia and failure to thrive despite medical treatment.

Palliative surgery—banding the pulmonary artery   Until recently, banding the pulmonary artery was the usual operation for infants with a large ventricular septal defect who remained in heart failure in spite of medical treatment. At operation, the pulmonary artery is partially occluded, so reducing pulmonary blood flow. The procedure usually allows the infant to leave hospital, but often with a reduced exercise tolerance, the possibility of increasing cyanosis, and sometimes a continued need for digoxin and diuretics. There is a risk of right to left shunting if the band is applied too tightly or if acquired infundibular stenosis develops, and there is still a risk of pulmonary vascular disease if the band is too loose. The combined mortality from banding and later total correction is about 20%. The results of early total correction of ventricular septal defects are now better than this in some centres, and in these circumstances banding is seldom performed for an uncomplicated VSD. It is still required for complex lesions in which there is an increased pulmonary blood flow, but which are not suitable for early correction (for example, an atrioventricular canal with a high pulmonary flow).

    The pulmonary artery is approached through a left thoracotomy and a thick ligature is threaded around it. Systemic and pulmonary arterial pressures are monitored, the former obtained directly from the aorta or from a peripheral artery cannulated at the start of the operation, while the pulmonary arterial pressure distal to the site of banding is generally measured via a needle inserted through its wall. These pressure measurements are critical to the success of the operation, and it is essential to ensure that the child is well ventilated when they are made. Ideally, the band is tightened progressively until the pulmonary arterial pressure falls to normal (30 mm Hg; 4·0 kPa). The systemic pressure increases slightly at the same time. An alternative technique is to tighten the band until the rise in systemic arterial pressure reaches a plateau.

    It is important to appreciate that banding the pulmonary artery imposes a considerable strain on the right ventricle and predisposes to right to left shunting. Occasionally, the child's condition deteriorates 10 to 15 minutes after the band has been applied, and it is therefore wise to monitor the arterial pressure and heart rate with particular care at this stage. The pulmonary arterial pressure proximal and distal to the band, and the systemic pressure and oxygen tension are measured before the chest is closed to ensure that optimum haemodynamic conditions have been achieved.

Corrective surgery Early closure of uncomplicated ventricular septal defects is being advocated with increasing frequency for the reasons given above. Management during and after surgery follows the general principles outlined on p. 166, and the operative procedure and its sequelae are similar to those described in Chapter 7.

Prolonged respiratory difficulties are common following both palliative and corrective surgery for ventricular septal defect. Long periods of controlled ventilation may be required, and a maintained positive airway pressure is often helpful, but care must be taken to prevent pulmonary damage caused by the use of large tidal volumes and high ventilatory pressures.

The tetralogy of Fallot

The mean age of survival of children with untreated tetralogy of Fallot is 12 years. The creation of an anastomosis between the pulmonary artery and a systemic vessel increases blood flow through the lungs and improves arterial oxygenation. This leads to a reduction in polycythaemia and its thrombotic complications. Survival is significantly improved, but the long-term results of palliative surgery still reveal a mortality of between 20 and 40% after 20 years with possibly less than 10% of survivors remaining in comfortable health. At the present time, total correction between the ages of 1 and 4 years seems to offer the chance of substantial improvement on these results, long-term figures suggesting that late mortality is small and that most survivors are symptom-free. However, very long-term figures are not available yet. The difficulty at present is to decide whether to offer early total correction to the infant whose condition is deteriorating, or to perform a palliative procedure with total correction later. The combined mortality of palliation and later correction is 25–30%, whereas a mortality of less than 10% for early total correction has been reported from some experienced centres.

A palliative procedure is still selected if the anatomical conditions are unfavourable (in particular, if the pulmonary artery is very small), and aorto-pulmonary shunts are also used to relieve more complex cardiac lesions in which the pulmonary blood flow is reduced. Transventricular pulmonary valvotomy, performed as a closed procedure, is only undertaken occasionally now as a first stage operation for the tetralogy of Fallot.

Palliative procedures—the Blalock and Waterston shunt operations The Waterston shunt, a side-to-side anastomosis between the ascending aorta and pulmonary artery, is carried out from the right side of the chest. The Blalock anastomosis can be performed from either side and consists of an end-to-side anastomosis between the subclavian artery and the corresponding pulmonary artery. The blood supply to the arm is derived thereafter from anastomoses around the scapula, but decreased growth in the limb is sometimes visible. Intra-arterial pressure monitoring is valuable but not essential in these sick infants, but the cannula must be placed in a vessel in the opposite arm if a Blalock shunt is to be created.

Cyanosis and polycythaemia are common preoperatively. Although the polycythaemia is a physiological response to prolonged hypoxaemia, it increases the peripheral vascular resistance and increases the chance of thrombotic complications. If the operation is successful, the hypoxaemic stimulus to haemopoiesis will diminish, and it is therefore reasonable to attempt to reduce the haematocrit during surgery by replacing blood loss with plasma. It is also important to avoid dehydration.

Ventilation with high concentrations of oxygen will do little to relieve the systemic desaturation although 50% oxygen in nitrous oxide is widely advocated to minimise hypoxaemia caused by pulmonary collapse during thoracotomy. Circulatory collapse is rare during operation unless the side clamps on the aorta or main pulmonary artery are placed too far across the vessel, so impeding blood flow through it. Haemorrhage is sometimes a problem after the anastomosis has been completed, but if the operation is straightforward, the infant's condition is often good at the end of surgery and controlled ventilation is only required if the cardiac output remains poor or the child is cold. Occasionally too large a shunt is created and pulmonary oedema develops. This is sometimes of such severity that controlled ventilation is required, or even reoperation to narrow the shunt.

Total correction of the tetralogy of Fallot Total correction at an early age eliminates some of the problems encountered if the operation is delayed until later. Adhesions following previous surgery are not present, bronchial collateral vessels are less well developed and there is no question of an aortopulmonary shunt requiring closure or control before bypass can be established.

The operation itself is often straightforward and follows the course described in Chapter 7. Postoperative problems are common, particularly respiratory insufficiency. Passage of a normal blood flow through the underdeveloped pulmonary circulation, elevation of the left atrial pressure, and damage inflicted by the entry of particulate material directly into the lungs during bypass via bronchopulmonary collaterals may all contribute. Heart block, myocardial failure and haematological disturbances are also common and are discussed in more detail in Chapter 7.

Transposition of the great arteries

In this condition, one of the most common causes of cyanotic heart disease in infancy, the aorta arises from the right ventricle and the pulmonary artery from the left. Oxygen can only reach the systemic circulation by communications between the left and right heart such as through a patent foramen ovale, septal defect or patent ductus arteriosus. Without treatment, 85 to 90% of these children die before the age of 1 year. Balloon septostomy, the creation of an atrial septal defect at cardiac catheterisation by withdrawing an inflated balloon through the foramen ovale, markedly improves the chances of survival because it provides better mixing of oxygenated (pulmonary) and deoxygenated (systemic blood) at atrial level. If corrective surgery is delayed too long, however, progressive arterial hypoxaemia occurs and no more than 50% of children will survive beyond the age of 2 years.

Palliative surgery   Rashkind's balloon septostomy provides good immediate palliation and is now performed at the initial catheterisation on all infants with transposition of the great arteries, irrespective of associated lesions. After the age of 3 months, and in some cases of transposition with multiple associated lesions, the results of balloon septostomy are unsatisfactory and an atrial septal perforation has to be created surgically (Blalock-Hanlon operation).

   This procedure entails considerable interference with the circulation and carries a high mortality. Two techniques are commonly employed; in the first, the right pulmonary artery and veins are snared, and a clamp is placed on the right atrial wall near the interatrial groove in such a way that part of the septum is included in the clamp. The atrium is opened and a portion of septum is excised. The atrial clamp is then partially released, allowing the septum to slip out of it, and the clamp is quickly reapplied. The pulmonary snares can then be released and the atrial incision closed.

   An alternative technique consists of snaring both superior and inferior venae cavae. The heart is allowed to empty for a few beats, and then it is either fibrillated or an aortic clamp is applied. The empty heart can then be opened through the right atrium, a portion of septum excised, and the atrial wall clamped for closure within 3 minutes from the onset of caval obstruction. Profound bradycardia is almost inevitable during this manœuvre, and if the heart stops spontaneously, resuscitation is often unsuccessful. The results are improved if a syringeful of the infant's own blood is drawn up before the heart is opened, and is used to fill the atrium as soon as it has been closed. In this way, the heart is not presented immediately with a bolus of stored blood which is hypoxic, acidotic and hyperkalaemic. Whichever technique of septectomy is chosen, emergency action to restore a satisfactory heart action is often needed. Myocardial stimulants such as isoprenaline, adrenaline and calcium chloride must be ready in suitable dilution together with warmed blood for transfusion and sodium bicarbonate to correct metabolic acidosis. A small dose of bicarbonate is sometimes given immediately before the septectomy is performed. Ventilation with 100% oxygen for 3 or 4 minutes before the procedure and again as soon as the circulation is restored may minimise the chance of dysrhythmias or cardiac arrest.

Corrective surgery Transposition of the great arteries carries a high mortality in spite of palliative procedures and there is a considerable morbidity from thromboembolic episodes. Early correction is favoured now, usually when the child is between 6 and 18 months of age.

Anatomical correction is only feasible occasionally, but physiological correction is usually possible by means of the Mustard operation which is carried out with the aid of cardiopulmonary bypass. There is considerable variation in the cardiac anatomy in cases of transposition and terminology is complex. However, the principle of the operation is that a 'baffle' of pericardium is introduced into the atria in such a way that the systemic venous return is directed into the left ventricle which supplies the pulmonary artery, while pulmonary venous blood is directed into the right ventricle which gives origin to the aorta. When the pericardium is scarred from previous surgery, a baffle of woven Dacron can be used instead.

The results of surgery depend on whether or not the baffle achieves complete separation of the systemic and pulmonary venous drainage and whether or not its presence causes any degree of systemic venous obstruction. Passage of some blood through the baffle is possible in the first few hours after insertion if it is made of a synthetic material; arterial hypoxaemia can therefore persist for a short time, but full saturation should be achieved within 6 hours of surgery.

When left ventricular outflow tract obstruction occurs in conjunction with transposition of the great arteries, it can either be relieved through the pulmonary artery or left ventricle, or, in severe cases, a conduit can be inserted between the left ventricle and pulmonary artery. If pulmonary hypertension has developed in a patient with transposition of the great arteries and a ventricular septal defect, a palliative Mustard operation is performed and the septal defect is left patent.

The operation designed by Rastelli is undertaken as an alternative to the Mustard procedure in patients with transposition of the great arteries, ventricular septal defect and pulmonary stenosis. A conduit is inserted from the right ventricle to the main pulmonary artery to replace the stenosed pulmonary outflow tract which is ligated. The ventricular septal defect is repaired in such a way that left ventricular blood is directed through it into the aorta.

Total anomalous pulmonary venous drainage

Although this lesion accounts for only 1·5% of congenital heart disease, it has a mortality of about 80% in the first year of life. The pulmonary veins drain into the right side of the heart through a communicating channel which may be above or below the diaphragm. These infants are cyanosed and often suffer from gross pulmonary oedema. There is no satisfactory palliative treatment, and complete correction must be attempted as soon as the diagnosis has been established in symptomatic infants, or if there is pulmonary hypertension. At operation, the common pulmonary veins are anastomosed to the back of the left atrium and the communicating channel is usually closed. During surgery, intermittent obstruction to the pulmonary veins can cause considerable variation in pulmonary compliance and hence in the efficiency of gas exchange.

Aortic stenosis

Corrective surgery provides the only chance of survival for infants with severe heart failure from aortic stenosis. Open valvotomy is performed, either on cardiopulmonary bypass or using profound hypothermia and circulatory arrest, but it is rarely possible to leave a normally functioning valve because the cusps are thick and non-compliant. Poor left ventricular function is common and it is sometimes difficult to decide whether this is due to left ventricular failure or to endocardial fibroelastosis.

Aorto-pulmonary window

Infants with an aorto-pulmonary window are at risk from two main complications: severe heart failure and the early development of pulmonary vascular disease. Transaortic patch closure is commonly regarded as the easiest and safest operative procedure.

Persistent truncus arteriosus

This is a complex defect in which there is no continuity between the right ventricle and pulmonary artery. The ventricles communicate through a septal defect, and a common vessel, the truncus arteriosus, supplies both the pulmonary and systemic circulations. The natural history of this lesion is unfavourable: without operation, 80% of patients will die during the first year of life and survivors are likely to develop pulmonary vascular disease. Banding the pulmonary artery offers some palliation although the mortality is high and the technical difficulties of subsequent total correction are increased. Physiological correction can be achieved by inserting a valved conduit between the right ventricle and the pulmonary arteries. Most surgeons favour this approach, rather than palliation in infancy, even though the conduit may require replacement as the child grows.

Atrioventricular canal

Partial and complete forms of this anomaly are recognised. When the defect is incomplete, there is a primum atrial septal defect (p. 121) associated with anatomical abnormalities of the atrioventricular valves. In more severe cases, the atrioventricular valves are incompetent, and when there is a total atrioventricular canal, there is also communication across the ventricular septum.

Partial forms of the condition rarely cause heart failure in infancy although if this does occur, total correction should be performed. Pulmonary artery banding has been used in the past to treat complete atrioventricular canal in infancy, but the mortality has been high because of atrioventricular valve incompetence. Recently there have been encouraging reports of early total correction.

Pulmonary atresia

1 With intact ventricular septum   Most attempts at total correction of this lesion in infancy have failed. Palliation can sometimes be achieved by closed pulmonary valvotomy and creation of a systemic to pulmonary arterial shunt.
2 With ventricular septal defect   These patients often remain asymptomatic for several years with right to left shunting through the septal defect and pulmonary blood flow derived from systemic collateral arteries. If this flow becomes too great and cardiac failure develops, some of the collaterals can be ligated. Occasionally this lesion causes severe cyanosis in infancy in which case the creation of a systemic to pulmonary arterial shunt should be considered.

Cor triatriatum

A barely perforate septum divides the left atrium into two chambers. Patients with this condition present in infancy with heart failure and pulmonary oedema caused by obstruction to pulmonary venous drainage. Complete recovery follows excision of the septum.

The procedures outlined in this chapter can only be performed satisfactorily in centres equipped to deal with infants. At present, total correction in infancy is generally preferred for lesions such as total anomalous pulmonary venous drainage, aortic or pulmonary stenosis and aorto-pulmonary window, and may be advisable for ventricular septal defect, the tetralogy of Fallot and transposition of the great arteries, particularly if the infant's condition is deteriorating. Palliation is indicated for some defects, for example, pulmonary atresia, and may be preferable for the conditions listed above if facilities for open heart surgery in infancy are not available. Neither palliation nor correction is justified in centres which lack the necessary facilities and expertise for dealing with infants with congenital heart disease, and attempts to treat occasional cases are rarely successful.

REFERENCES

GENERAL PRINCIPLES

Leading Article (1975) Congenital heart disease: incidence and aetiology. *Lancet* **2**, 692.
PANG L. M. & MELLINS R. B. (1975) Neonatal cardiorespiratory physiology. *Anesthesiology* **43**, 171.

DIAGNOSTIC PROCEDURES

STRANGER P., HEYMANN M. A., TARNOFF H., HOFFMAN J. I. E. & RUDOLPH A. M. (1974) Complications of cardiac catheterisation of neonates, infants and children—a three year study. *Circulation* **50**, 595.

ASPECTS OF GENERAL ANAESTHETIC MANAGEMENT

BENNETT E. J., RAMAMURTHY S., DALAL F. Y. & SALEM M. R. (1975) Pancuronium and the neonate. *British Journal of Anaesthesia* **47**, 75.
GOUDSOUZIAN N. G., MORRIS R. H. & RYAN J. F. (1973) The effects of a warming blanket on the maintenance of body temperature in anesthetized infants and children. *Anesthesiology* **39**, 351.
MIYASAKA K., EDMONDS J. F. & CONN A. W. (1976) Complications of radial artery lines in the paediatric patient. *Canadian Anaesthetists' Society Journal* **23**, 9.

CARDIAC SURGERY IN INFANCY

BAILEY L. L., TAKEUCHI Y., WILLIAMS W. G., TRUSLER G. A. & MUSTARD W. T. (1976) Surgical management of congenital cardiovascular anomalies with the use of profound hypothermia and circulatory arrest. Analysis of 180 consecutive cases. *Journal of Thoracic and Cardiovascular Surgery* **71**, 485.
BARRATT-BOYES B. G., SIMPSON M. & NEUTZE J. M. (1971) Intracardiac surgery in neonates and infants using deep hypothermia with surface cooling and limited cardiopulmonary bypass. *Circulation* **43**, 44.
EDMUNDS L. H., GREGORY G. A., HEYMAN M. A., KITTERMAN J. A., RUDOLPH A. M. & TOOLEY W. H. (1973) Surgical closure of the ductus arteriosus in premature infants. *Circulation* **48**, 856.
JOHNSTON A. E., RADDE I. C., STEWARD D. J. & TAYLOR J. (1974) Acid-base and electrolyte changes in infants undergoing profound hypothermia for surgical correction of congenital heart defects. *Canadian Anaesthetists' Society Journal* **21**, 23.
KIRKLIN J. W. (1973) *Advances in Cardiovascular Surgery*. Grune and Stratton, New York.

SEELYE E. R., HARRIS E. A., SQUIRE A. W. & BARRATT-BOYES B. G. (1971) Metabolic effects of deep hypothermia and circulatory arrest in infants during cardiac surgery. *British Journal of Anaesthesia* **43**, 449.

STARK J. (1976) Debate on congenital heart disease: early total repair is preferable to palliative surgery. *Advances in Cardiology* **17**, 51.

POSTOPERATIVE MANAGEMENT

COGSWELL J. J., HATCH D. J., KERR A. A. & TAYLOR B. (1975) Effects of continuous positive airway pressure on the lung mechanics of babies after operation for congenital heart disease. *Archives of Diseases of Childhood* **50**, 799.

GREGORY G. E., EDMUNDS L. H., KETTERMAN J. A., PHIBBS R. H. & TOOLEY W. H., (1975) Continuous positive airway pressure and pulmonary and circulatory function after cardiac surgery in infants less than three months of age. *Anesthesiology* **43**, 426.

HATCH D. J., COGSWELL J. J., TAYLOR B. W., BATTERSBY E. F., GLOVER W. J. & KERR A. A. (1973) Continuous positive airway pressure after open heart operations in infancy. *Lancet* **2**, 469.

CHAPTER 10

COMPLICATIONS OF OPEN HEART SURGERY

Mechanical hazards
Systemic embolism
Haemorrhage and coagulation disorders
Reversal of specific coagulation defects
Jaundice
Cardiac tamponade; the 'cardiac compression syndrome'

Pulmonary damage
Cerebral damage
Renal failure
'Low output syndrome'

There are hazards associated with open heart surgery and cardiopulmonary bypass which can complicate operative or postoperative management. This chapter includes a general account of the main problems; some have been discussed in more detail in earlier chapters, but they are considered again here for the sake of completeness.

MECHANICAL HAZARDS

Equipment failure is now rare and pumps or disc oxygenators can be operated manually in the event of a power failure. Defective components in the circuit present a greater problem but can generally be changed quickly. It may be necessary to discontinue perfusion for a few minutes but this rarely results in significant tissue damage, particularly if the interruption occurs during a hypothermic perfusion. Even a relatively slight reduction in body temperature (e.g. to 33°C) provides considerable protection. The most serious hazard is clot formation in the extracorporeal circuit. This either causes complete obstruction, generally in the filter, or if perfusion is still possible, clot is disseminated throughout the body. The control of coagulation is discussed on pp. 84 and 88.

Vascular damage can occur when the great vessels are cannulated. Well recognised complications include dissection of the wall of the femoral artery (p. 136), obstruction to, or exclusive perfusion of the innominate artery if blood is returned to the aorta (p. 137), and damage to the ostia of coronary arteries (p. 137) leading to occlusion and myocardial ischaemia. Occasionally, it is difficult to repair the aorta or femoral artery after the cannula has been removed; a false aneurysm develops postoperatively in a few cases and may require further surgery.

SYSTEMIC EMBOLISM

Systemic embolism is inevitable if coagulation takes place in the extracorporeal circuit, but it can also occur in more subtle ways. Particulate material accumulates within the apparatus because clot, calcium, vegetations or fat are returned from the heart and pericardial cavity; platelet and white cell aggregates develop intravascularly or are present in stored blood added during perfusion, and denatured proteins accumulate as a result of damage in the oxygenator. Most of this debris is removed by efficient filtration (p. 141), but some reaches the patient. Microemboli can be identified during perfusion using special techniques of ultrasonic monitoring of the arterial return which enable particulate material to be distinguished from air bubbles, and emboli can also be demonstrated at post mortem by histological examination. Silicone antifoam used in the oxygenator was a prominent cause of systemic embolism at one time, but technical improvements and the introduction of new materials have greatly reduced the importance of this hazard.

Ultrasonic monitoring also reveals gas bubbles in the blood returned to the patient. The importance of this is difficult to assess because the number of patients at risk as judged by ultrasonic monitoring is greatly in excess of the number who show evidence of embolic damage. A possible explanation is that the bubbles are largely composed of oxygen and carbon dioxide rather than of air, and are therefore easily reabsorbed. The incidence of gaseous embolism depends on the selection of equipment, the design of the circuit and the flow rates of both blood and gas. The formation of gas bubbles is virtually impossible in a membrane oxygenator unless the membrane is punctured, whereas the incidence rises with bubble oxygenators as the flow rates of both blood and fresh gas are increased. Excessive flow rates and fast rotation of the discs increase the risks of gaseous embolism from disc oxygenators. Bubbles can also be generated at points of high negative pressure, and sharp angles or sudden changes of diameter which encourage the formation of eddies must be eliminated. Occasionally gas bubbles are liberated from solution by overrapid heating.

Another cause of systemic embolism is air introduced into the left heart at the time of operation. This is notoriously difficult to eliminate, especially from a dilated, poorly contracting ventricle. It can be prevented from reaching the systemic circulation during perfusion by aortic cross-clamping or by inducing ventricular fibrillation, but there is always a risk that some will reach the cerebral or coronary vessels when the heart beat is restored and the aortic clamp is removed. Before perfusion is discontinued, efforts are made to eliminate air through the vent by lifting the heart out of the pericardium so that the left ventricular apex is the highest point. Gentle artificial ventilation of the lungs at this stage helps to drive air out of the pulmonary veins. A needle is often inserted subsequently into the highest point on the aorta so that any residual air can be eliminated here when the ventricle starts to eject. Attempts to reduce the danger of air embolism by flooding the operative field with carbon dioxide, which is highly soluble in blood, are rarely successful because it diffuses into the atmosphere too readily. Similarly, although there is a theoretical danger that the effects of air embolism will be enhanced by the inert gas effect when nitrous oxide is restarted, changes in anaesthetic technique are rarely implemented on this basis, perhaps because it is difficult to determine if significant air embolism has occurred.

The significance of embolic damage in general is difficult to assess. There are measurable defects in the function of most organs postoperatively, but the damage is often non-specific and emboli cannot be identified in every case which comes to post mortem. Differences in perfusion technique can be related to different degrees of organ dysfunction and may reflect the incidence of microembolism; membrane oxygenators, haemodilution and small pore filters have all been shown to be advantageous, and it remains to be seen whether further improvements can be made in the design of extracorporeal apparatus.

HAEMORRHAGE AND COAGULATION DISORDERS

Serious haemorrhage is one of the most common complications of open heart surgery. Factors which increase the incidence of bleeding are pericardial adhesions from disease or previous surgery, dilated, thin-walled cardiac chambers or great vessels, and operations in the presence of sepsis or recent myocardial infarction. Sometimes haemorrhage occurs from a single site where sutures tear out repeatedly. Alternatively, bleeding continues slowly from every raw surface. Coagulation defects are often present and should be suspected if there is generalised bleeding or if no clot is formed after the usual dose of protamine has been given.

The control of haemorrhage depends upon adequate access to the source of bleeding, the reversal of specific coagulation defects, and empirical treatment with transfusions of fresh blood, platelets or fresh frozen plasma. It is sometimes difficult to identify the source of bleeding, particularly if the tissues are distorted during attempts to locate it. The site may be difficult to reach, for example if haemorrhage is occurring from the back of the aorta, and sometimes access is only possible at the expense of such distortion of the heart that the cardiac output falls or dysrhythmias occur. Even when the site of bleeding can be reached easily, repair may be difficult because friable tissues fail to hold sutures well or because the intravascular pressure is so high that the sutures tear out before the repair is complete.

Transfusion must be continued to maintain an optimal blood volume as far as possible but the atrial pressures are difficult to interpret while the heart is being distorted. Dysrhythmias and hypotension caused by disturbance to the heart may embarrass the circulation to such an extent that it is wiser to improve access by extending the incision. A median sternotomy can be extended by a laterally directed thoracotomy which provides access to the left ventricle. This means that the left pleural cavity will be widely opened and will require drainage at the end of the operation, but ventilation should remain undisturbed.

The technique of inflow occlusion is used occasionally, particularly if the aorta cannot be repaired easily because the high intraluminal pressure causes individual sutures to tear out. Inflow occlusion entails a short period of circulatory arrest which must be timed very carefully. The snares around the cavae are tightened so that these vessels are completely occluded. After a few beats, the heart is virtually empty and the aorta is then cross-clamped beyond the site of bleeding. Sutures can be inserted in the flaccid aortic wall, and because each one does not tear out as soon as it has been inserted, it is often possible to complete the repair within the two or three minutes of circulatory arrest which can be tolerated. The manœuvre is obviously dangerous. It should be preceded by a few breaths of 100% oxygen, and cardiosupportive drugs should be ready to give if an adequate circulation fails to return as soon as the aortic clamp and caval snares have been removed. The only reassuring feature of the technique is that the coronary vessels are, at least theoretically, being supplied with oxygen by blood which enters the heart through the coronary sinus and passes through the lungs in the usual way.

Reversal of specific coagulation defects

Coagulation mechanisms may be impaired preoperatively in patients with cyanotic congenital heart disease or those who have been treated with anticoagulants. Large doses of heparin are given during perfusion, and heparin reversal with protamine is often carried out empirically. The platelet count is always depressed during bypass and some degree of fibrinolysis occurs, even in uncomplicated cases. Coagulation defects may be associated with the use of excessive doses of dextran, and coagulation factors can be diluted by massive transfusions of stored blood which is deficient in a number of these factors. Abnormal coagulation can be induced *in vivo* by haemorrhage or circulatory failure, and excessive fibrinolysis may develop subsequently.

The term 'heparin rebound' is used to describe failure of coagulation recurring after clot has once been formed. It may occur because large volumes of heparinised blood have been transfused from the oxygenator without the administration of additional protamine, or because an improved blood supply has swept heparinised blood out of tissues which were previously poorly perfused, or because sulphases in blood destroy the heparin/protamine complexes. An excess of protamine can itself produce coagulation defects, but even if no measured indication for protamine exists, a small increment (100 mg) can be given without harm. In practice, protamine deficiency is an uncommon cause of serious haemorrhage in the postperfusion period.

If fibrinolysis is suspected, the *in vitro* clot lysis time can be used as an index of severity. Dissolution of clot at 37°C in less than 60 minutes indicates that significant fibrinolytic activity exists, and times of less than 20 minutes indicate severe fibrinolysis. If fibrinolysis persists unchecked, the fibrinogen content of blood falls and the titre of circulating fibrin degradation products rises, but the time required to complete these estimations is such that they are only of real value when haemorrhage is persistent but not massive.

Aprotinin (Trasylol) and ε-aminocaproic acid are both directly antifibrinolytic and also interfere with the synthesis of fibrinolysin. ε-aminocaproic acid is sometimes given prophylactically during perfusion and either drug may be used after perfusion if fibrinolysis is suspected or proven. The dose of aprotinin is 100 000 units initially followed by 50 000 units every hour until haemorrhage stops; rapid intravenous injection can cause hypotension. If ε-aminocaproic acid is chosen, an initial dose of 100 mg/kg is given intravenously and the same amount can be repeated every 4 hours. It too can cause hypotension if injected rapidly, and it accumulates if the urine output is low because excretion is through the kidneys. Excess antifibrinolytic therapy can promote pathological degrees of intravascular thrombosis, and proof of its efficacy in the control of haemorrhage after open heart surgery is poor.

Calcium depletion is a theoretical cause of coagulation defects if large volumes of ACD or CPD blood have been transfused rapidly, particularly if citrate metabolism is impaired by hypothermia or circulatory failure. If calcium salts are considered necessary, calcium gluconate is preferable to the chloride because it is less likely to provoke ventricular ectopic beats or ventricular overactivity: 10 ml of 10% calcium gluconate (2·25 mmol calcium) are given by slow intravenous injection.

Vitamin K is given to patients who have been treated preoperatively with coumarin-type anticoagulants, but the mechanism and time course of its action are such that immediate benefit cannot be expected.

Fresh blood and fresh frozen plasma both contain a rich supply of intrinsic coagulation factors. Fresh blood supplies viable platelets too if it is transfused within 4 hours of collection, whereas the advantage of fresh frozen plasma is that it is available more readily. Isolated coagulation defects rarely occur after cardiopulmonary bypass, and empirical transfusion with fresh blood or fresh frozen plasma (20 ml/kg) is often the most successful treatment. Platelet transfusions are also effective although, in theory, do not replace all the absent coagulation factors. Obvious sources of heavy bleeding should be secured before fresh blood, plasma, or platelets are given.

JAUNDICE

There is inevitably some haemolysis and blood destruction after massive transfusions. Jaundice may appear postoperatively and is more likely to occur if the liver was engorged preoperatively or has been damaged by a prolonged period of circulatory insufficiency. The biochemical picture is rarely one of pure haemolysis, and evidence of hepatocellular dysfunction is generally prominent. Jaundice later in the postoperative period is more likely to be due to infection, either endocarditis or wound sepsis; jaundice occurring 3 to 6 weeks after operation is often caused by infection with cytomegalovirus, and later still Australia antigen positive hepatitis may be responsible. Haemolytic jaundice in the late postoperative period can result from blood damage on prosthetic valves, particularly if there is a paraprosthetic leak.

CARDIAC TAMPONADE; THE 'CARDIAC COMPRESSION SYNDROME'

Blood loss continues in the postoperative period, but drainage of more than 200 ml/hour is excessive and may indicate that the patient should be returned to the theatre for further attempts at haemostasis. Normally the chest drains are kept on suction and the tubing is 'milked' with rollers to express blood clot and prevent blood accumulating in the pericardial space. If these measures are unsuccessful, the heart is compressed by liquid blood or by clot and a condition which is analogous to cardiac tamponade develops. The physical signs may differ from those seen when a tense pericardial effusion has developed more slowly (p. 64). In the first place, blood loss from the circulation is occurring simultaneously. This tends to lower the venous pressure while blood accumulating around the heart causes the venous pressures to rise. Secondly, a systolic descent in the atrial waveform, which is characteristic of a pericardial effusion, will be eliminated if there is regurgitation across the atrioventricular valves. Thirdly, clot may accumulate around only part of the heart, and the typical haemodynamic changes do not develop even though some of the chambers are compressed. Finally, it may be difficult to detect the usual physical signs in patients who are established on artificial ventilation. Dyspnoea is less apparent, although the patient may 'fight the ventilator', and it is generally impossible to detect pulsus paradoxus.

Cardiac compression is particularly likely to occur if there is heavy blood loss which drains intermittently, and the diagnosis cannot be excluded merely because the pericardial sac was not closed completely at operation. The characteristic signs are progressive elevation of the atrial pressures, often in spite of blood loss, while the systolic and pulse pressures fall. The peripheral circulation is constricted, the patient is restless and the urine output falls early.

Elevation of the atrial pressures must be distinguished from overtransfusion, but it is the distinction from worsening myocardial failure which is most difficult. The chest X-ray is of little help because the heart shadow often looks enlarged immediately after operation and the mediastinum is commonly widened. If there is any doubt, it is wiser to reopen the chest and it may be safer to do this in the Intensive Care Unit to prevent the disturbance of movement. Anaesthesia with 50% nitrous oxide in oxygen is generally all that is required. A non-depolarising muscle relaxant can be given to ensure control of ventilation, and small doses of diazepam (2·5 mg) or papaveretum (2·5–5 mg) may be necessary if the patient has not reached the stage of critical circulatory failure.

If tamponade is present, circulatory function improves as soon as the chest is open. Slight improvement may also occur if a grossly distended, failing heart is decompressed by opening the sternum or pericardium, but this improvement is likely to be short-lived. A further search is made for the source of bleeding after blood and clot has been removed from the pericardial sac, but quite often an individual bleeding point cannot be identified. Coagulation mechanisms should be reviewed at the same time, particularly if there is slow oozing from all surfaces of the wound.

PULMONARY DAMAGE

The nebulous term 'pump lung' dates from the early days of open heart surgery when unexplained pulmonary dysfunction was a prominent cause of postoperative morbidity and mortality. Use of the term has tended to persist even though it is now rare to see florid pulmonary damage which cannot be clearly related to an identifiable cause.

Many factors can interfere with the lungs after cardiac surgery. Chest wall movement is limited by pain, lateral thoracotomy causing greater mechanical impairment than median sternotomy. Bronchial secretions can accumulate during prolonged anaesthesia, particularly if humidification has been inadequate or if there is bronchial hypersecretion associated with heart failure. Episodes of left atrial hypertension cause alveolar damage, although frank pulmonary oedema is unlikely unless the left atrial pressure remains elevated, and debris from stored blood may contribute if small pore filters have not been used. In addition, there does appear to be a specific element of pulmonary pathology related solely to cardiopulmonary bypass. Histological examination of lung biopsies taken at the end of perfusion reveals damage to both capillary endothelium and alveolar epithelium. White cells and platelets of abnormal appearance are trapped within the pulmonary capillaries and there is degranulation of mast cells. Physiological studies carried out postoperatively on patients who have never shown signs of heart failure demonstrate an increase in the alveolar-arterial oxygen tension gradient and in the dead space/tidal volume ratio. These changes are maximal at 48 hours and decrease slowly thereafter.

Pulmonary damage during bypass has been attributed to the release of lysosomal enzymes and vasoactive substances, and there is some evidence that pretreatment with large doses of methyl prednisolone affords protection. However, corticosteroid therapy does not appear to influence the physiological derangements described above, possibly because other factors which are not steroid sensitive also contribute.

The pulmonary damage which occurs with modern techniques of cardiopulmonary bypass does not present a serious hazard to the majority of patients. If, however, pulmonary function is deranged for other reasons, or if the circulation is compromised and cannot sustain the work of breathing, relatively minor degrees of pulmonary damage can be critical. The incidence of pulmonary complications is minimised by careful monitoring and control of the left atrial pressure, by the use of haemodilution rather than whole blood during perfusion, and by ensuring that both the arterial return and blood transfused intravenously are filtered effectively. Pretreatment with methyl prednisolone (30 mg/kg) may be desirable in high risk cases.

Prolonged ventilation is occasionally necessary after open heart surgery, but in the absence of circulatory complications, most patients can resume spontaneous ventilation within 3 to 36 hours.

CEREBRAL DAMAGE

Measurable defects of psychological and intellectual function occur in more than 50% of patients following cardiopulmonary bypass, but the incidence of gross deficits is very much smaller and only a few patients are left with a permanent disability. Factors which increase the risk of cerebral damage are advancing age, prolonged perfusion and the presence preoperatively of cerebral or cerebrovascular disease.

The brain can be damaged by particulate or gaseous emboli, or by inadequate cerebral perfusion. Monitoring cerebral electrical activity reveals that the onset of bypass is a time of particular hazard although changes can occur at other times. Signs of cerebral damage should be sought postoperatively with particular care if there are abnormalities on the EEG or Cerebral Function Monitor during perfusion, although the magnitude of the lesion cannot be predicted accurately in many cases. Neurological signs are likely to deteriorate over the first 48 hours and minor signs are, in any case, easy to miss immediately after operation. If cerebral damage has occurred, it is wise to continue controlled ventilation to diminish the risks of hypoxaemia, hypercarbia, or elevation of the venous pressure. Symptomatic measures are often required to control hyperthermia or convulsions, and corticosteroids are generally given to limit the development of cerebral oedema. Dexamethosone is widely considered to be the steroid of choice, 10 mg stat and 4 mg every 6 hours thereafter.

Measures which reduce the incidence of cerebral damage include the use of small pore filters on the arterial return, prompt treatment of hypotension, the avoidance of hypocapnia or sudden changes in blood temperature, and careful elimination of air from the left heart at the end of bypass.

RENAL FAILURE

Formerly a common complication of open heart surgery, renal failure is now rare. It is almost always caused by a prolonged period of renal ischaemia associated with circulatory failure rather than by any disturbance associated with cardiopulmonary bypass.

'LOW OUTPUT SYNDROME'

This term is used to describe multisystem failure occurring after open heart surgery as the result of a prolonged period of circulatory insufficiency. The most common cause is myocardial failure, often present to some extent pre-operatively but exacerbated during or after operation by overdistension, dysrhythmias, prolonged ischaemia, or coronary arterial damage or embolism. Other causes include incomplete correction of the cardiac abnormality, the development of a leak around a prosthetic valve or intracardiac patch, or the physical size of a valve prosthesis within the ventricular cavity. Dysfunction of a prosthetic valve and unrecognised cardiac compression from blood clot are occasional causes.

Pulmonary dysfunction is inevitable and requires prolonged intermittent positive pressure ventilation. The urinary output is negligible, jaundice develops in a few days and there is persistent paralytic ileus. Consciousness may be present initially but ultimately the patient is comatose.

Signs of circulatory failure are manifest—the atrial pressures are always elevated because transfusion is continued to exclude the possibility of hypovolaemia. The heart rate is often unremarkable because both rhythm and rate are generally amenable to control. The blood pressure is low and the pulse pressure generally very low, although if inotropic agents with peripheral vasodilating properties are used, the diminution in pulse pressure and degree of peripheral vasoconstriction are less extreme than might be anticipated in the presence of the other features. Peripheral gangrene is uncommon for the same reason.

Therapy is based on three principles: the exclusion of treatable causes, pharmacological or mechanical support for the failing circulation, and specific measures to control individual organ failure. The details of management are beyond the scope of this book and the reader is referred to texts on postoperative intensive care.

REFERENCES

MECHANICAL COMPLICATIONS

BULKLEY B. H. & ROBERTS W. C. (1974) Isolated coronary arterial dissection. A complication of cardiac operations. *Journal of Thoracic and Cardiovascular Surgery* **67**, 148.

MAGNER J. B. (1971) Complications of aortic cannulation for open heart surgery. *Thorax* **26**, 172.

SALAMA F. D. & BLESOVSKY A. (1970) Complications of cannulation of the ascending aorta for open heart surgery. *Thorax* **25**, 604.

TAYLOR P. C., GROVES L. K., LOOP F. D. & EFFLER D. B. (1976) Cannulation of the ascending aorta for cardiopulmonary bypass: experience with 9000 cases. *Journal of Thoracic and Cardiovascular Surgery* **71**, 255.

EMBOLISM

BASS R. M. & LONGMORE D. B. (1969) Cerebral damage during open heart surgery. *Nature* **222**, 30.

CONNELL R. S., PAGE U. S., BARTLEY T. D., BIGELOW J. C. & WEBB M. C. (1973) The effect on pulmonary ultrastructure of Dacron wool filtration during cardiopulmonary bypass. *Annals of Thoracic Surgery* **15**, 217.

GALLAGHER E. G. & PEARSON D. T. (1973) Ultrasonic identification of sources of gaseous microemboli during open heart surgery. *Thorax* **28**, 295.

HILL J. D. (1973) Blood filtration during extracorporeal circulation. *Annals of Thoracic Surgery* **15**, 313.

LAWRENCE G. H., McKAY H. A. & SHERENSKY R. T. (1971) Effective measures in the prevention of intra-operative aero-embolus. *Journal of Thoracic and Cardiovascular Surgery* **62**, 731.

WRIGHT G. & SANDERSON J. M. (1976) Cellular aggregation and destruction during blood circulation and oxygenation. *Thorax* **31**, 405.

HAEMORRHAGE AND COAGULATION DISORDERS

BACHMANN F., McKENNA R., COLE E. R. & NAJAFI H. (1975) The hemostatic mechanisms after open heart surgery. I: studies on plasma coagulation factors and fibrinolysis in 512 patients after extracorporeal circulation. *Journal of Thoracic and Cardiovascular Surgery* **70**, 76.

BOYD A. D., ENGELMAN R. M., BEAUDET R. L. & LACKNER H. (1972) Disseminated intravascular coagulation following extracorporeal circulation. *Journal of Thoracic and Cardiovascular Surgery* **64**, 685.

GRALNICK H. R. & FISCHER R. D. (1971) The hemostatic response to open heart operations. *Journal of Thoracic and Cardiovascular Surgery* **61**, 909.

INGLIS T. C. McN., BREEZE G. R., STUART J., AGRAMS L. D., ROBERTS K. D. & SINGH S. P. (1975) Excess intravascular coagulation complicating low cardiac output. *Journal of Clinical Pathology* **28**, 1.

McCLURE P. D. & IZSAK J. (1974) The use of epsilon-aminocaproic acid to reduce bleeding during cardiac bypass in children with congenital heart disease. *Anesthesiology* **40**, 604.

McKENNA R., BACHMAN F., WHITTAKER B., GILSON J. R. & WEINBERG M. Jr. (1975) The hemostatic mechanism after open heart surgery. II: frequency of abnormal platelet functions during and after extracorporeal circulation. *Journal of Thoracic and Cardiovascular Surgery* **70**, 299.

PLIAM M. B., McGOON D. W. & TARHAN S. (1975) Failure of transfusion of autologous whole blood to reduce banked requirements in open heart surgical patients. *Journal of Thoracic and Cardiovascular Surgery* **70**, 338.

WAGSTAFFE J. G., CLARKE A. D. & JACKSON P. W. (1972) Reduction of blood loss by restoration of platelet levels using fresh autologous blood after cardiopulmonary bypass. *Thorax* **27**, 410.

JAUNDICE

AHMAD R., MANOHITHARAJAH S. M., DEVERALL P. B. & WATSON D. A. (1976) Chronic hemolysis following mitral valve replacement: a comparative study of the Bjork-Shiley, composite-seat Starr-Edwards, and frame-mounted aortic homograft valves. *Journal of Thoracic and Cardiovascular Surgery* **71**, 212.

LOCKEY E., COSSART Y. & GONZALES-LAVIN L. (1973) Serum hepatitis after open heart surgery. *Thorax* **28**, 188.

SINGH H. M. & BARKER J. T. (1974) Jaundice following open heart surgery. *Thorax* **29**, 68.

SLATER S. D., SALLAM I. A., BAIN W. H., TURNER M. A. & LAWRIE T. D. V. (1974) Haemolysis with Bjork-Shiley and Starr-Edwards prosthetic heart valves: a comparative study. *Thorax* **29**, 624.

CARDIAC TAMPONADE

CUNNINGHAM J. N. Jr., SPENCER F. C., ZEFF R., WILLIAMS C. D., CUKINGNAN R. & MULLIN M. (1975) The influence of primary closure of the pericardium after open heart surgery on the frequency of tamponade, post-cardiotomy syndrome and pulmonary complications. *Journal of Thoracic and Cardiovascular Surgery* **70**, 119

CEREBRAL, PULMONARY AND RENAL DAMAGE

ABEL R. A., BUCKLEY M. J., AUSTEN W. G., BARNETT G. O., BECK C. H. Jr. & FISCHER J. E. (1976) Etiology, incidence, and prognosis of renal failure following cardiac operation: results of a prospective analysis of 500 consecutive patients. *Journal of Thoracic and Cardiovascular Surgery* **71**, 323.

ABERG T. (1974) Effect of open heart surgery on intellectual function. *Scandinavian Journal of Thoracic and Cardiovascular Surgery Supplementum* **15**.

BEVAN D. R., BIRD B., LUMLEY J. & NORMAN J. (1973) Fluid loading and cardiopulmonary bypass: a study of renal function. *Anaesthesia* **28**, 631.

Leading Article (1975) Brain damage after open heart surgery. *Lancet* **2**, 399.

LLAMAS R. & FORTHMAN H. J. (1973) Respiratory distress syndrome in the adult after cardiopulmonary bypass. *Journal of the American Medical Association* **225,** 1183.

PARKER D. J. (1975) Some changes in the lungs associated with cardiopulmonary bypass (p. 459). In *Lung Metabolism,* Ed. A. F. Junod & R. de Haller. Academic Press, London.

VEITH F. J., HAGSTROM J. W., PANOSSIAN A., NEILSEN S. L. & WILSON J. W. (1968) Pulmonary microcirculatory response to shock, transfusion, and pump-oxygenator procedures. A unified mechanism underlying pulmonary damage. *Surgery* **64,** 95.

LOW OUTPUT STATE AND POSTOPERATIVE CARE

BRAIMBRIDGE M. V. & BRANTHWAITE M. A. (1972) *Postoperative Cardiac Intensive Care,* 2nd Edition. Blackwell Scientific Publications, Oxford.

INDEX

195

MAR 1 0 1978

Dr. & Mrs. A. Z. Guanzon
1329 ARLINGTON AVENUE
SASKATOON, SASK.
S7H 2Y1